Sleeping Soundly

Sleeping Soundly

UNDERSTANDING AND TREATING SLEEP DISORDERS

Dr Antonio Ambrogetti

ALLEN & UNWIN

Acknowledgement
Figures 21 and 23 are reproduced from: Fell, D. 1995 'Screening of truck drivers for sleep apnoea in New South Wales: potential road safety benefit' in *Staysafe 28: Sleep Disorders, Driver Fatigue and Safe Driving*, First Report of the Joint Standing Committee on Road Safety of the 51st Parliament, Parliament of New South Wales, pp. 83–103.

First published 2000

Allen & Unwin
83 Alexander Street
Crows Nest NSW 2065
Australia
Phone: (61 2) 8425 0100
Fax: (61 2) 9906 2218
Email: info@allenandunwin.com
Web: http://www.allenandunwin.com

National Library of Australia
Cataloguing-in-Publication entry:

Ambrogetti, Antonio, 1952– .
  Sleeping soundly: understanding and treating sleep disorders.

  Includes bibliography.
  Includes index.
  ISBN 1 86508 372 0

  1. Sleep disorders. 2. Sleep disorders—Treatment. 3. Insomnia
  4. Insomnia—Treatment. 5. Sleep—Physiological aspects.
  I. Title.

616.8498

Set in 11/19 pt Sabon by DOCUPRO, Canberra
Printed by Griffin Press Pty Limited, Adelaide

10 9 8 7 6 5 4 3 2

To my parents, and for Bronwyn, Robert and Toni

Foreword

Dr Ambrogetti's book is a welcome addition to the literature on sleep. It provides a valuable interface between media articles and detailed textbooks. Why we sleep remains a mystery. Much has been learnt by the study of sleep disorders.

Disorders of sleep have been around for many years but knowledge about them has been accelerated by modern technology. It is quite likely that modern civilisation has increased the number of sleep disorders. In particular, our ability and need to work 24 hours per day together with our enthusiasms for food (leading to obesity) and for various drugs (leading to disturbances during sleep) have produced problems with sleep that are highly significant for our society.

In this book, Dr Ambrogetti provides for a broad range of readers a superb summary of the disorders of sleep and a thoughtful introduction to how they might be managed. The strength of this approach is that in a relatively brief book the reader finds information that will provide both understanding and insight into one or more sleep problems that may be affecting them or their family.

The more common sleep problems, especially insomnia, sleep apnoea and out of phase body clock syndrome, are covered in particular detail. Other sections address less common problems.

In addition there is a personal approach to sleep problems in children. The investigation of sleep disorders is highlighted, especially its contribution to understanding, by those suffering from sleep problems.

Michael J. Hensley MB BS PhD FRACP FAFPHM
Professor of Medicine
The University of Newcastle

Director Department of Respiratory and Sleep Medicine
John Hunter Hospital

Contents

Foreword   vii

Preface   xi

1 An overview of sleep   1

2 How sleep is measured   18

3 Snoring and disturbed breathing   28

4 Body jerks and restless limbs   45

5 Insomnia   59

6 Sleepiness, tiredness and fatigue   85

7 Children and sleep   108

8 Medications and sleep   129

9 Sleep disorders and driving   142

10 Dreams and dreaming   149

Appendix 1: Sleep-related internet sites   175

Appendix 2: International sleep organisations   177

Appendix 3: Sleep centres and support groups in
    Australasia   179

Appendix 4: The function of sleep   183

Further reading   186

Glossary   193

Preface

The field of sleep medicine has seen an enormous progress in knowledge and understanding over the last forty years. Sophisticated monitoring and imaging techniques have given us detailed insight into the nature of sleep and an understanding of its derangement. In fact, the last *International Classification of Sleep Disorders* (1990) lists 88 sleep disorders. At the same time, the advent of multimedia technology and the internet has made available to the public a large—at times, overwhelming—amount of information. It is not easy to distinguish information that reflects well-proven facts from unsubstantiated statements and hypotheses yet to be proven. This book originates from clinical practice. It is not intended to be an exhaustive source of information on sleep; rather, it tries to integrate specific knowledge with practical sleep problems.

The first two chapters give an overview of sleep and provide useful basic information. The other chapters deal with specific problems. Issues that are specific to childhood are discussed in Chapter 7. Dreams and dreaming is a topic of great interest, raising issues not only of medicine but also psychology, religion and philosophy. Some aspects of dreaming are reviewed in Chapter 10.

An important concept emphasised throughout the book is

that *sleep* is part of the *sleep and wake* function. For cultural reasons we think of sleep and wakefulness as separate entities. In fact, sleep and wake are part of a single function that lasts 24 hours and it is attuned to the light and dark cycle. There are important implications to the notion of sleep and wake. The first is that symptoms of sleep disturbances often manifest themselves during the day, even though the origin of the problem is at night. The connection between nighttime problems and daytime symptoms is often not made or very delayed. The second is that to improve sleep quality it is often necessary to modify our daytime behaviour rather than changing our nighttime routine or taking sleeping tablets.

I hope that this book is of help to people who are interested in exploring sleep in its multiple aspects.

I would like to thank Karla McCormack, journalist with the Marketing and Media Services of the University of Newcastle for her help.

I am indebted to the Royal Newcastle Sleep Disorders Centre where I have worked for the last ten years with many people with sleep disorders. I am grateful to my secretaries, Therese Benson and Amanda Holliday, for preparing this manuscript. I would also like to thank Lyndal Hayward and Annette Barlow from Allen & Unwin for their enthusiastic support and helpful suggestions.

Antonio Ambrogetti
MD, FRACP

1

An overview of sleep

- Sleep should be looked at in terms of both sleep and wake function, not just nighttime.
- Sleep is different in different people.
- The way you function during the day is as important to good sleep quality as good sleep is to your daytime function.
- Sleep structure and quantity change with age.
- The human body can cope with sleep deprivation for a long time, and symptoms of lack of sleep may only become apparent after months or years of chronic sleep deprivation.

Before we can properly understand sleep disorders and how best to treat them, we need to understand what sleep is, and how sleep and wake are related.

✳ What is sleep?

Although everyone knows what sleep is, it is difficult to define. Sleep is a state of the body which can be recognised by:

- immobility (the person is more still than when they are awake);

- special body position (people fall asleep in a preferred position); and
- the ability to fully wake up if stimulated. (This is different from people who are unconscious.)

What is 'normal' sleep?

Defining normal sleep is difficult, because everyone has their own sleep pattern. For practical purposes we will consider a 'normal' sleep to be the sleep of people without a sleep complaint.

❋ How are sleep and wake related?

There is a part of the brain called the brain stem which operates roughly on a 24-hour cycle, promoting sleep during part of the cycle and wakefulness during the other. We will refer to this centre as the *sleep–wake centre* (Figure 1). This centre is a poorly defined network of neurones (cells of the nervous system) connected to each other in a complex interaction. It is closely related to other functions that are not under our direct control. These functions are regulated by the autonomic nervous system. Blood pressure, pulse rate, kidney function, digestion, sweating and hormone secretion are a few examples of bodily functions that are regulated independently of our will. The same area of the brain also regulates other important aspects of our daily living, such as emotions, memory and concentration. It should come as no surprise, then, that disruption of the sleep and wake function is often associated with somatic (body) and mental symptoms such as muscle ache and

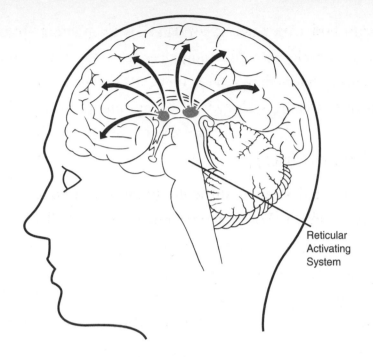

Figure 1   Sleep–wake centre

pain, nausea, poor memory and concentration, irritability and mood changes, to mention a few.

✳ What influences sleep and wake?

Sleep is different in different people

How much sleep people need, and how well they sleep, varies from person to person according to their genetic make up. This is true for all people, whether or not they have sleep problems. Although most people sleep for seven to eight hours, some sleep much less (short sleepers) or much more (long sleepers). There are documented cases of people sleeping for less than two hours per day for many years. These people are able to function well during the day with little sleep. There is no obvious difference between short sleepers and long sleepers in how cheerful they are or how much they can achieve. Whether a person feels they have had enough sleep varies from one person to another. This topic, and the effects of lack of sleep, are discussed in more detail in Chapter 6.

Sleep and wake affect each other

Sleep and wake are interlinked because they are part of the same function. Anything that disturbs sleep will disturb wakefulness, and vice versa. People say that if they 'could just get a good night's sleep' they would feel much better during the day. The opposite is also true: if you function well during the day, your sleep will also be of good quality. Because sleep and wake cannot be separated, the treatment of some sleep disorders involves changing what a person does during the day so that they sleep better at night. Sleep disorders associated with depression and anxiety, chronic fatigue and insomnia are all disorders whose treatment should be aimed at modifying daytime function as much as nighttime habits.

Light and darkness cycle

Light and darkness are very important in making the sleep–wake centre in the brain work properly. The centre tunes the body to be awake when it is light, and asleep when it is dark. This worked very well when people did not have artificial light, and when they worked during daylight and rested at night. Now that we have artificial light and can be working at any hour, it is easy for the body to become confused about when it should be awake and when it should be asleep. However, while artificial light may have created some sleep problems, it can also be used to help correct them. Natural light can also be useful for treating some sleep and wake disorders (see Chapter 5).

Biological rhythms

Many body functions, both in humans and animals, are regulated by biological rhythms. Some are well known, such as hibernation which can last for months and allows certain animals to survive the hardships of winter. Others are very short, lasting minutes and sometimes seconds. Examples are hormone secretion, respiration and heart rate. The rhythm that is of particular importance to sleep is the *circadian rhythm*, which lasts approximately 24 hours (circa-diem = about a day).

The area of the brain where the biological clock is situated is called the *suprachiasmatic nucleus*. It is located near the sleep–wake centre (Figure 2). Sleep and wake is tightly synchronised with two other functions, body temperature and melatonin secretion, which have their own rhythm. The action of synchronising functions together is technically referred to as *entrainment*.

The suprachiasmatic nucleus can be considered a form of 'master clock' which has an internal timer of about 24 hours. To be precise, the timer varies slightly, from one person to another, between 23 and 27 hours. It is entrained primarily

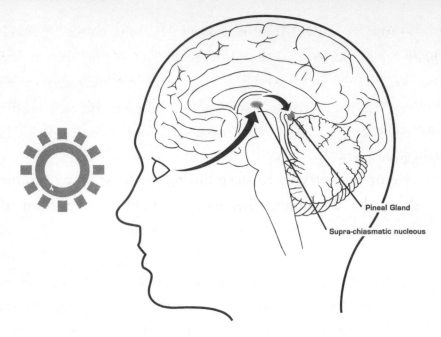

Pineal Gland

Supra-chiasmatic nucleous

Figure 2   Position of the biological clock in the brain

by the light and darkness cycle. As shown in Figure 2, during daytime, when light activates the retina in the back of the eye, a tiny signal is transmitted through the optic nerve to the suprachiasmatic nucleus. When light is present the suprachiasmatic nucleus tends to suppress the secretion of melatonin in the body. At nighttime, *and* with darkness, the opposite happens: the melatonin is released and its level rises in the blood. In the morning, with bright light, the cycle starts again.

Body temperature, measured as internal body temperature, also has a 24-hour rhythm that is synchronised with the 'body clock'. In fact, body temperature has been the easiest way to study the circadian clock. Our tendency to fall asleep is maximal at the time the body temperature is low, between 11 p.m.

and 4 a.m. and from 2 p.m. to 4 p.m. The mid-afternoon sleep tendency, the 'siesta' of the Latino-American, reflects this body tendency. It occurs irrespective of food intake. By the same token, alertness peaks in the morning and late afternoon. These observations are important in understanding why a night worker who sleeps during the day does not obtain good-quality sleep. He or she is trying to sleep during the most unfavourable period of the 24 hours. Sleeping at night is important if refreshing and restoring sleep is to be obtained.

Medical conditions and medications

Medical problems can interfere with sleep and daytime function. Some illnesses can keep people awake at night—for example, illnesses where the person is in a lot of pain or has symptoms that can disrupt sleep, such as the coughing and wheezing of asthma.

Medications can also affect sleep and wake. For example, antihistamines, used for allergies and contained in over-the-counter medicines for the 'flu, can make the person sleepy during the day. Others, such as cortisone and bronchodilators for asthma, have a stimulant effect and can keep the person awake at night.

Internal and external events

Internal events, things happening within our body, can affect sleep and wake. If a person has a painful condition—for example, arthritis or a broken arm—this will affect the way they operate during the day as well as disturbing their sleep at night. Thoughts and feelings are also internal events that may affect a person's sleep and wake. If someone is under constant mental stress, their performance and sense of well-being can drop during the day and they may not sleep as well at night. This is often the case in chronic depression and anxiety disorders.

External events, things that happen outside the body, can also affect sleep and wake. A noisy environment or an uncomfortable bed can affect the amount of sleep a person gets and how well they sleep.

Diet and exercise

Many other factors can affect the sleep–wake centre. The regularity of bedtime and wake-up time is very important in training the sleep–wake centre. The more regular these activities are, the better. The same applies to regular mealtimes and exercise.

The question of how diet influences sleep remains a controversial, if popular, topic. It is often said that a diet rich in carbohydrates and fat increases sleepiness. This theory is based on a small number of subjects studied in experimental conditions, and sleepiness was self-reported. In fact, the time of day when meals are taken may have more to do with sleepiness than the meals themselves. For example, sleepiness is increased after midday and evening meals, but not after breakfast. The effect of diet on sleep quality is small, if present at all.

Another contentious issue is the effect of exercise on sleep. It is often said that vigorous exercise should be avoided in the evening because it increases wakefulness and so has a negative effect on sleep. However, the evidence for this is scanty. Studies in both normal sedentary subjects and athletes show no significant deterioration in sleep quality following moderate or vigorous exercise.

So, should a person exercise at night? The answer comes from what we have just said and common sense. If someone wakes up at 5.30 a.m. to go to work and returns home at 8 p.m., two hours of exercise in the gym is likely to be detrimental. In this situation the problem is not the exercise itself, but the fact that resting and sleep time is affected. Apart from this, there appears to be no strong reason not to exercise in the evening.

Age

The amount of time spent asleep and awake in every 24 hours changes through life (Figure 3). In a foetus a regular cycle of activity and rest is recognised at about 30–32 weeks of pregnancy. A newborn baby spends about sixteen hours a day asleep. The average time spent asleep in every 24 hours falls from sixteen hours in a baby, to seven to eight hours in adulthood, and to six hours or less in old age. As life progresses, the kind of sleep we get changes as well as how long we sleep. However, contrary to common belief, the 'need for sleep' does not decrease with age. The amount of light sleep increases with age. Older people are more likely to have illnesses, and so the number of awakenings also increases, causing more disrupted sleep and poorer sleep quality.

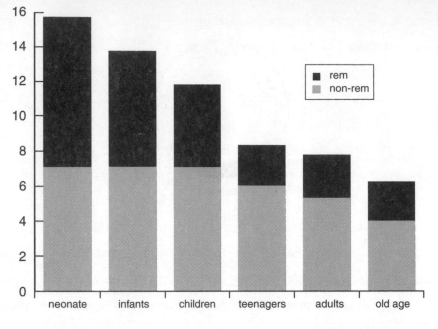

Figure 3 The amount of sleep decreases through life (data from Roffwarg *et al, Science* 1966, vol. 156, pp. 604–19)

Daylight saving

Daylight saving was initially introduced as an energy-saving strategy and has been adopted in many industrialised countries. In spring the clock is moved forward, causing the loss of one hour, and in autumn the reverse happens with one hour gained. The effect of daylight saving on sleep among a group of people in the south of England during the autumn change was studied in the 1970s by Timothy Monk and Simon Folkard. They showed that it takes five to six days for complete adaptation to daylight saving to occur. People kept waking earlier than the new legal time, suggesting that the 'internal clock' adjusts slowly and is sensitive to even minor changes.

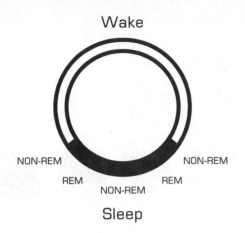

**Figure 4   24 hours sleep and wake cycle, approximately
2/3 awake 1/3 asleep**

It could be anticipated that even more disruption occurs in
spring when there is a loss of one hour.

✳ Sleep is an active process

The discovery in the late 1940s of a system that actively maintains wakefulness (the reticular activating system—Figure 1)
reinforced the popular belief that sleep was a passive event.
It was thought that when the part of the brain that is active
during wakefulness switches off, our body goes to sleep. This
was in keeping with the simple view of sleep as a resting period
for the body to recover for the following day. However, experiments in animals and observations in humans have shown that
sleep is an *active* process. Growth hormone secretion and cell
division are increased during sleep. The destruction of certain
parts of the brain can result in complete lack of sleep. Stimulation of other parts makes sleep more likely to occur. This

suggests that certain parts of the brain are active during sleep. The recording of the electrical activity of the brain has taught us that sleep is a complex and active state of the body.

Brain activity during sleep

For as long as people have been sleeping, we have been intrigued by sleep. However, it was only in the first half of the twentieth century that brain waves were first recorded using the electroencephalogram (EEG), allowing more insight into the functioning of the brain. Based on the EEG, sleep and wake function shows a regular pattern over a 24-hour period (Figure 4). If we measure brain waves, eye movements and muscle tone, it is possible to identify the brain's different states of activity (Figure 5).

✳ Wakefulness

Wakefulness occupies approximately two-thirds of a 24-hour period and is a complex state during which our performance is affected by many factors. Sometimes a person can be wide-awake and at other times very drowsy. The quality and intensity of external stimuli conveyed by our senses, and internal stimuli (our thoughts and feelings) affect our functioning during wakefulness. For example, if something is interesting, our concentration and attention span are activated, producing an overall increase in alertness. In a boring situation, such as driving at a constant speed on a highway, some people find that their level of alertness decreases and they struggle to stay awake. In these situations, involuntary episodes of sleep

Wake

Non-REM sleep

stage
1

2

3-4

REM sleep

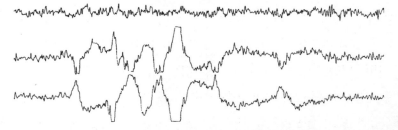

Figure 5 **During sleep the brain is very active with different electrical waves. In REM there are periods of eye movement.**

can occur during wakefulness. These episodes are called *microsleeps*.

Microsleeps (daydreaming)

The ability to record brain waves continuously for 24 hours has allowed us to identify very brief periods of sleep that intrude during wakefulness. Microsleeps, during which the person is momentarily 'absent' from the events around them, are not noticeable just by observing a person's behaviour. To others, the person seems awake but 'daydreaming' or 'disinterested'. That person is virtually sleeping with their eyes open.

❋ REM and non-REM sleep

Measuring the eye movements and muscle tone during sleep has allowed the identification of two different sleep states: rapid eye movement (REM) sleep and non-REM sleep.

REM sleep

Rapid eye movement was initially reported by George Trumbull Ladd in 1892. However, the importance of REM sleep was established by Dr Eugene Aserinsky and Nathaniel Kleitman in the early 1950s when studying children's sleep. It attracted people's attention, because it was initially thought to be closely associated with dreaming. It is now accepted that dreams occur during both REM sleep and non-REM sleep (see Chapter 9).

An important feature of REM sleep is the almost complete lack of muscle tone (muscle power). If, for some reason, muscle power is maintained during REM the person can have abnormal behaviour during sleep, such as acting out their dreams. (See 'REM behaviour disorder', Chapter 4.)

Non-REM sleep

In normal conditions, sleep starts in non-REM sleep. The brain waves slow down and there are slow, rolling eye movements. Depending on the size and speed of the brain waves, non-REM sleep has been artificially divided into four stages: stages 1, 2, 3 and 4. This is currently the way that sleep is described.

During sleep, a person moves through the non-REM and REM sleep cycle five to six times each night. Periods of REM sleep tend to last longer in the second part of the night. The amount of non-REM and REM sleep changes through life, with REM sleep representing approximately 40–50 per cent of sleep at birth and approximately 20–25 per cent in adulthood and later ages.

'Early to bed early to rise, make a man healthy, wealthy and wise.'

This quotation, repeated generation by generation and credited to Benjamin Franklin, has no scientific basis. It is a convenient excuse for sending children to bed early, to give their parents some peace and quiet. However, there is no evidence that 'larks' (early-to-bed people) are more healthy or wealthy or wise than 'owls' (late-to-bed people).

✳ The effects of sleep deprivation

Sleep deprivation, not enough sleep, is very common in our society and is perhaps the most frequent cause of fatigue,

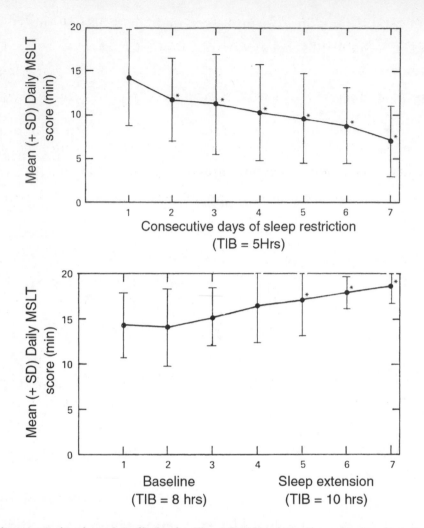

Figures 6 (top) and 7 (below) The 'y' axis plots the minutes it takes to fall asleep. The smaller the number, the sleepier the person. TIB = time in bed. (Republished with permission of the American Sleep Disorders Association 'Nocturnal determinants of daytime sleepiness' M.A. Carskadon & W.C. Dement, *Sleep*, vol. 5, 1982)

tiredness and daytime sleepiness. Figure 6 shows the effect of reducing nighttime sleep to five hours for seven days. The numbers in the vertical axis are a measure of sleep tendency during the day. (The lower the number, the faster the person falls asleep or the sleepier he or she is.)

As we can see, the person becomes progressively more sleepy because sleep deficit accumulates over time. Conversely, extra time in bed in the morning can increase the level of alertness (Figure 7).

Here the study subjects slept for their usual eight hours for the first three nights. On the following four nights, they were allowed an extra two hours in bed and their level of alertness increased. (They were less sleepy during the day.) Studies such as these indicate that even a minor reduction in the amount of sleep has an effect on the way we function. However, because our body has a large function reserve, we can tolerate sleep deprivation for a long time, sometimes years, before symptoms appear.

2

How sleep is measured

- A careful account of what a person does during the day is a very important part of assessing sleep disorders.
- A self-reported sleep diary gives the patient a better insight into his or her sleep habits.
- Laboratory measurement of sleep length and structure at nighttime, and of sleepiness during the day, is sometimes needed for accurate assessment of sleep and wake function problems.

❋ Investigations of sleep and wake function

There are several methods that doctors and other health professionals use to investigate the nature of a person's sleep and wake function. Some methods involve listening to the patient's description of their sleep and wake pattern (subjective measures). Other techniques include measuring a person's brain waves and other body functions while they are asleep, as well as during the day (objective measures).

Subjective measures

Interview

During the interview the doctor will ask questions not only about sleep habits but also about daytime activities. What the patient does during the day is very important to their sleep. It is often useful for a partner or a member of the family to be present to report aspects of sleep behaviour of which the patient may not be aware.

Questions regarding sleep as a child and aspects of upbringing are part of the interview. Sometimes a psychiatric assessment is recommended. This is often a difficult request, which may not be welcomed by the patient. However, psychiatrists and clinical psychologists are professionals with special expertise in probing the emotional part of our lives, which is very important in sleep and wake function disorders.

Sleep diary

The person is often asked to keep a record of their bedtime, how long it takes them to fall asleep, the number of awakenings through the night, any medications they take, the time they get up, and a personal assessment of how well they slept. The sleep diary should be filled in when the person gets up in the morning. If they forget to fill in the diary after waking up, they should not fill it in later during the day because it can be difficult to remember how they slept. The sleep diary is usually kept for a week or two (see Figure 8).

Sleep questionnaire

There are many questionnaires used to measure subjective symptoms of sleepiness and disturbed sleep. A popular and simple one is the Epworth Sleepiness Scale (ESS), developed by Dr Murray Johns at the Epworth Sleep Disorder Centre in Melbourne. It measures the probability of falling asleep in a

Name:							Week: ____ to ____		
	Example	*Mon*	*Tue*	*Wed*	*Thur*	*Fri*	*Sat*	*Sun*	
1. I napped from ___ to ___ (note the times of all naps).	2.00 to 2.45 p.m.								
2 I took ___ mg of medication and/or ___ ml of ___ alcohol as a sleep aid.	ProSom 1 mg								
3. I went to bed at ___ o'clock and turned the light out at ___ o'clock.	10.30 11.15								
4. After turning the lights out, I fell asleep in ___ minutes.	45								
5. My sleep was interrupted ___ times (specify number of nighttime awakenings).	3								
6. My sleep was interrupted for ___ minutes (specify duration of each awakening).	20 30								
7. I woke up at ___ o'clock (note time of last awakening).	6.15								
8. I got out of bed at ___ o'clock (specify the time).	6.40								
9. When I got up this morning I felt ___ (1 = exhausted, 5 = refreshed).	2								
10. Overall, my sleep last night was ___. (1 = very restless, 5 = very sound).	1								

Source: C. Morin 1993 *Insomnia: Psychological Assessment and Management*, The Guilford Press, NY

Figure 8   Sleep diary

series of common daily situations (see Figure 9). The score on the ESS is between 0 and 24. Values above ten are suggestive of increased daytime sleepiness. However, there is poor correspondence between self-reported sleepiness and an objective measure of tendency to fall asleep, such as the multiple sleep latency test (discussed pp. 26–27).

Name: _____

Today's date: _____ Your age (years): _____

Your sex: (male = M; female = F): _____

How likely are you to doze off or fall asleep in the following situations, in contrast to feeling just tired? This refers to your usual way of life in recent times. Even if you have not done some of these things recently, try to work out how they would have affected you. Use the following scale to choose the most *appropriate number* for each situation:

0 = would *never* doze
1 = *slight* chance of dozing
2 = *moderate* chance of dozing
3 = *high* chance of dozing

Situation	*Chance of dozing*
Sitting and reading	
Watching TV	
Sitting, inactive in a public place (e.g. a theatre or a meeting)	
As a passenger in a car for an hour without a break	
Lying down to rest in the afternoon when circumstances permit	
Sitting and talking to someone	
Sitting quietly after a lunch without alcohol	
In a car, whilst stopped for a few minutes in the traffic	

Thank you for your cooperation

Figure 9 Epworth Sleepiness Scale (ESS). A score of over 10 is suggestive of increased sleepiness tendency. (Republished with permission of the American Sleep Disorders Association, 'A scale measuring daytime sleepiness' M. Johns, *Sleep*, 1991, vol. 6)

Objective measures

Overnight oximeter

An overnight oximeter is the recording of blood oxygen levels through the night. This test is used as a screening test for the

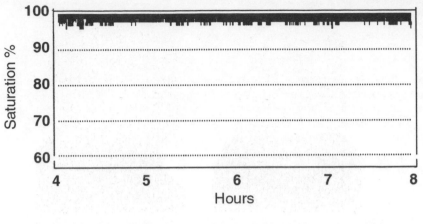

Figure 10   Normal oxygen level, above 90% and stable

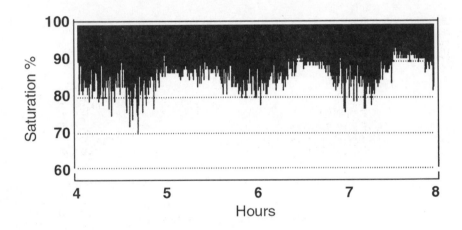

Figure 11   Sleep apnoea. The oxygen drops below the 90% level and there are continuous swings.

diagnosis of disturbed breathing during sleep (sleep apnoea). During sleep the level of oxygen is maintained unchanged by regular breathing. However, if the person has sleep apnoea the oxygen levels tend to fluctuate, and this suggests that a full sleep study is needed (Figures 10 and 11). The oximeter can be done in the patient's home with minimal disruption of their nighttime routine.

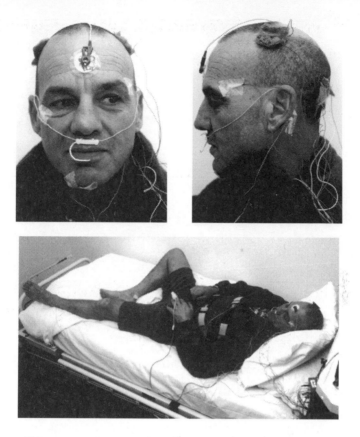

Figure 12   Preparation for an overnight recording

Overnight sleep study

An overnight sleep study is called *overnight polysomnography*.
(This term means 'graph of many sleep functions'.) During a
sleep study, a person attends the sleep unit in the evening and
is connected to wire leads (electrodes) before going to bed
(Figure 12). Different leads are applied to different areas to get
information about brain waves, eye movements, breathing,
blood oxygen, heart and muscle activity. This information is
recorded through the night under the supervision of a sleep
technician (Figure 13).

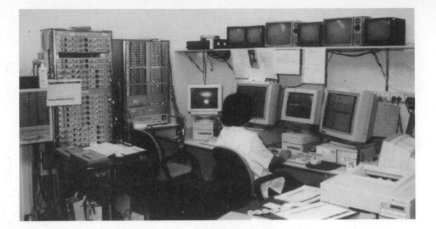

**Figure 13   Data from the patient is collected on computer CD
and analysed**

The overnight recording lasts about eight hours and is divided into thirty-second periods called *epochs* (Figure 14). Each study is composed of 700 to 960 epochs that are analysed (scored) individually by trained technicians. Polysomnography is a highly specialised and labour-intensive test. It provides information on the length and quality of sleep. It allows a measurement of how long it takes a person to fall asleep, and how many times they wake through the night. Microphones are often used to measure snoring, and elastic bands are applied to the chest to monitor the activity of the breathing muscles. Small gold-plated electrodes are applied to the shin to monitor leg movements, which are often seen in patients with restless legs (restless legs syndrome).

Because the person is not used to having wires attached to them and they are not sleeping in their own bed, the sleep is often somewhat different from at home. This is called the *first*

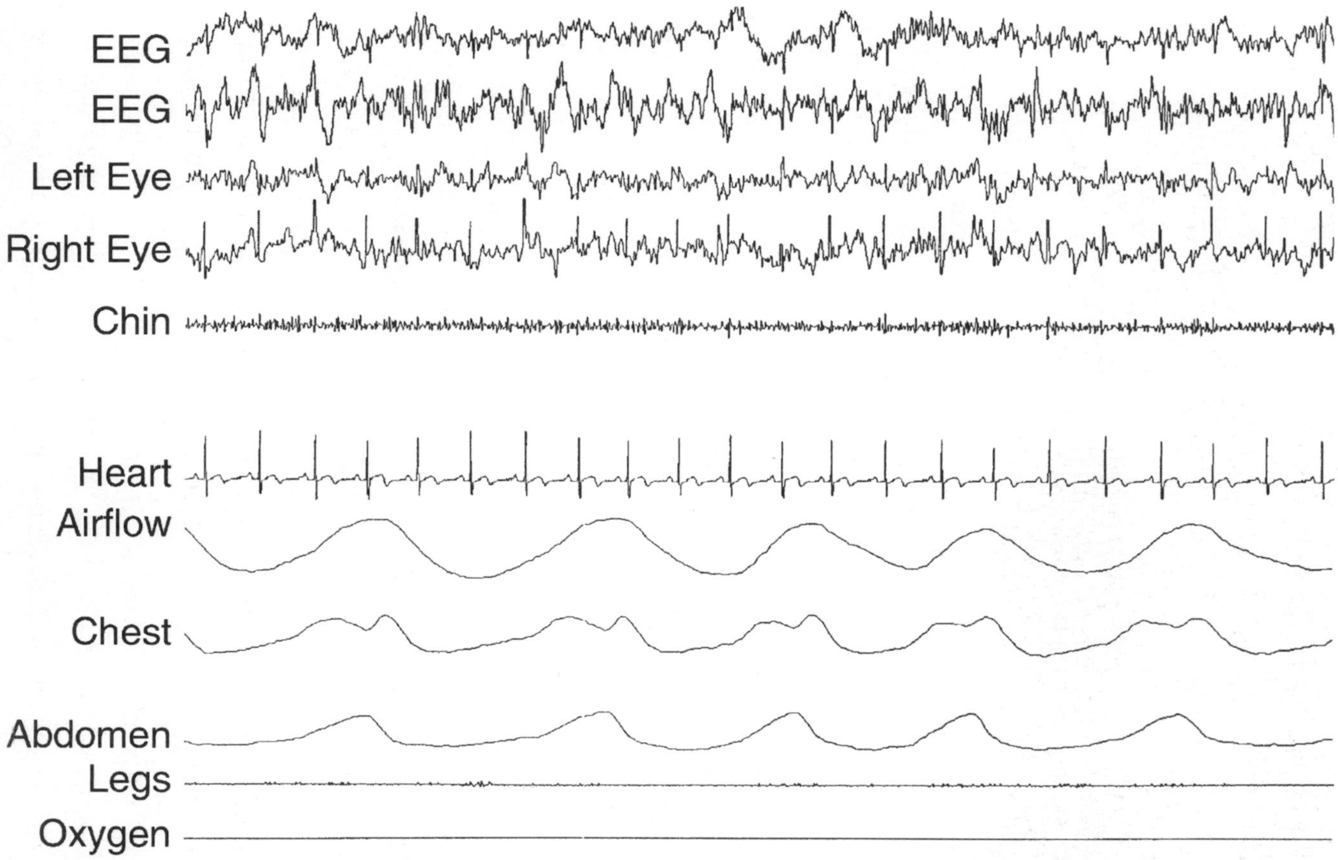

Figure 14 A thirty seconds recording (epoch) of sleep parameters. An overnight sleep study is about 700–800 epochs. Note that the airflow, chest and abdomen movements are regular and in phase.

night effect, and sometimes more than one night's re-cording is needed so that the person gets used to the procedure.

During the day before the sleep study the person should continue their usual routine unless special instructions are given. For example, they should have the usual amount of alcohol or coffee.

Multiple sleep latency test

After an overnight sleep study, some people may be required to stay at the sleep unit and have a test to find out how sleepy they are during the day. This test is called a *multiple sleep latency test* (MSLT). During an MSLT the person is allowed to have twenty-minute naps at two-hour intervals during the day. Typically the naps occur at about 9 a.m., 11 a.m., 1 p.m. and 3 p.m. The technicians at the sleep unit will measure how long it takes the person to fall asleep during each of the naps by observing changes in the brain waves recording.

Because the naps only last twenty minutes, only non-REM sleep is usually recorded. However, in some disorders such as narcolepsy, REM sleep can occur during these short naps and this can help in making a diagnosis.

A variant of the MSLT is called the *maintenance of wakefulness test*. In this test, the person is sitting in a comfortable chair in a darkened room and is asked to try and stay awake. The test lasts about forty-five minutes and is repeated throughout the day.

Assessment of the sleep–wake function requires a careful description of symptoms not only by the patient but also by family members because the patient may not be aware of abnormal events during sleep. Measuring sleep at nighttime and sleepiness tendency during the day is often required to define the problem with more precision.

3

Snoring and disturbed breathing

- Snoring and obstructive sleep apnoea are different.
- Snoring on its own is mostly a social problem.
- Weight reduction is usually the most important therapy.
- None of the available treatments—nCPAP, mouthguards and surgery—are 100 per cent effective.
- Symptoms of obstructive sleep apnoea are different in children and adults.

In this chapter we will discuss snoring and disturbed breathing during sleep, their significance, and why people are investigated and treated for these conditions.

✳ Breathing and sleep

In discussing breathing and sleep, the following definitions are useful:

- *Snoring.* Snoring is the noise produced by the air going through the throat while the person is asleep.
- *Apnoea.* Apnoea is a medical word for a condition where breathing stops *completely.*
- *Hypopnoea.* This is another medical word that refers to a condition where breathing stops *partially.* It is usually

defined as a 50 per cent decrease in breathing compared to breathing when awake.

When we fall asleep the body muscles tend to relax and become floppy, including the muscles in the back of the throat. As the air goes through, the floppy tissue vibrates and makes the noise of snoring. In some people the muscles become so floppy that they tend to collapse in the back of the throat, the air stops going through, and the person stops breathing completely (apnoea) or partially (hypopnoea). Stopping breathing can last from a fraction of a second up to 30 or 40 seconds or more.

✳ Snoring

Snoring is very common, with one in five people snoring almost every night. Men snore more than women, with a ratio of four to one. Women are also more likely than men to complain of the bed partner snoring.

Disturbed breathing during sleep is also common. Studies conducted among the general population in the Hunter Valley area of New South Wales suggest that at least one in every 25 people (4 per cent) have sleep apnoea. Similar results are found in other studies across the world.

Reason for investigating snoring

There are a few reasons why a person with snoring is investigated.

1 Snorers may disturb other people around them, even though they themselves are not disturbed by the problem. With few

exceptions, loud snoring is a problem not only because the patient makes the noise but also because the bed partner is a light sleeper. This is to say that, in these situations, snoring is a 'couple' problem where the snorer wears the brunt of the blame.

2 The bed partner has noticed that breathing stops and is concerned for the snorer's safety.

3 The person who is a snorer may wake up with a choking sensation, feel unrefreshed in the morning, and tired and sleepy during the day.

Treatment of snoring

The treatment of snoring includes general advice such as weight reduction, avoidance of alcohol in the two or three hours before going to bed, and the maintenance of clear nasal passages. If these manoeuvres are not sufficient, the use of a mouthguard can be effective in 60–70 per cent of cases.

Surgery to the palate, either with a scalpel or a laser beam (see Figure 17), is also an acceptable treatment with good results in 75–90 per cent of cases. However, when considering surgery for pure snoring, it should be remembered that treatment is undertaken for social reasons and not for strictly medical ones. There is no evidence that simple snoring causes short-term or long-term ill-health. The suggestion that snoring is a risk factor for high blood pressure needs to be proven. Surgery for snoring is quite different from, for example, surgery for an inflamed appendix where the surgery can be life-saving.

It should also be understood that surgery for snoring *is not a permanent cure.* As time passes, and in particular if a person puts on weight, snoring is likely to recur.

On occasions the choice to sleep in different rooms, because the husband or wife is a snorer, is a convenient excuse for not sleeping together. In this case, no treatment is effective or indicated.

✳ Obstructive sleep apnoea

Stopping breathing up to five times an hour, once every ten minutes on average, is unlikely to be harmful and is still considered normal. Stopping breathing completely more than five times an hour is called *obstructive sleep apnoea* (OSA) (or just *sleep apnoea*). If we consider both stopping breathing completely (apnoea) and partially (hypopnoea), the 'normal' limit is set at fifteen disturbed breathing periods an hour. The higher the number of disturbed breathing periods, the more severe the condition. By convention, stopping breathing fewer than thirty times an hour is considered mild and more than thirty, moderate to severe.

The term *Pickwickian syndrome* was used in the past to describe grossly overweight subjects with respiratory failure and daytime sleepiness. The majority had obstructive sleep apnoea and a decreased drive to breathe when awake.

Implications of sleep apnoea

During sleep apnoea, each time the person stops breathing the oxygen level in their blood starts falling and this fall in oxygen triggers the body to wake up. Sometimes the person will wake up completely, sometimes with choking feelings lasting a few seconds or a very dry mouth. However, the majority of the time the person does not wake up; instead, sleep becomes lighter, moving from deep stages to very superficial sleep, causing the person to be very restless.

These events account for the two most important consequences of sleep apnoea, which are poor sleep quality due to sleep fragmentation, and chronic lack of oxygen.

The most immediate consequence of disturbed breathing during sleep is sleep fragmentation. For example, if a person has stopped breathing thirty times an hour, their sleep tends to be disrupted that many times. The person wakes up unrefreshed, even if they have been asleep for ten hours, because sleep quality has been poor. They have increased tiredness and lethargy during the day. Their memory and concentration tend to deteriorate, and their mood can change, being moody, irritable or short-tempered. This, in turn, can cause personal, interpersonal and job-related problems. It is also reported that sexual drive and potency is reduced in patients with obstructive sleep apnoea.

It is important to realise that, although symptoms occur during the day, sleep apnoea occurs while the person is asleep and is often unaware of the problem. So, persons with sleep apnoea may be investigated and treated for chronic tiredness and fatigue or for depression, when the problem is actually sleep apnoea.

The other important consequence of disturbed breathing during sleep is chronic low oxygen at night. If the person stops breathing long enough, the oxygen drops below levels that are considered safe. If sleep apnoea continues undiagnosed and untreated for years, the person spends long periods with low oxygen in the body. Although not proven with certainty, obstructive sleep apnoea may carry an increased risk of cardiovascular diseases such as hypertension, heart attack and cerebrovascular accidents (stroke).

It has been suggested that chronic lack of oxygen due to sleep apnoea may be a cause of dementia. However, there is no evidence for this.

'Will my bed partner stop breathing and not start again?'

This is a frequently asked question and a major concern to many people attending our sleep centre. The answer is 'no'. When a person stops breathing and the oxygen drops to low levels, the body tends to wake the person and breathing starts again. It is surprising how the body can tolerate prolonged periods of low oxygen. The only possible situation when breathing may not restart is in some cases of sudden infant death syndrome (SIDS). However, even in this situation, evidence is not strong.

Risk factors for sleep apnoea

There are a number of factors that can increase the risk of having sleep apnoea. These factors are discussed below in order of importance.

Obesity

Increased weight is the most important risk factor for sleep apnoea. As you put on weight, snoring and stopping breathing increase, and vice versa. One possible explanation for this is

$$\frac{\text{BMI}}{\text{(Body mass index)}} = \frac{\text{weight (Kg)}}{\text{height}^2 \text{ (m)}}$$

Normal = 20–25

Overweight = 26–30

Obese = >30

Figure 15   Body mass index (weight is in kilograms and height in metres)

that fatty tissue can cause narrowing of the space in the throat. Together with obesity, a short and thick neck is often associated with sleep apnoea.

A good measure of obesity is the body mass index (BMI), which is calculated by dividing the weight in kilograms by the height in metres squared. Normal values are between 20 and 25; overweight is 26 to 30; and obesity is above 30 (Figure 15). A weight reduction of six to eight kilograms is often effective.

Alcohol and sedatives

Alcohol, like many sedative medications, is a muscle relaxant and can make the lining of the throat flaccid and, in turn, increase the risk of snoring and stopping breathing. It is common knowledge that if a person has a few drinks in the hours close to going to bed, they are likely to snore and to stop breathing more. Because the action of alcohol is short, usually two or three hours, the snoring and disturbed breathing are more obvious in the first part of the night. This effect of alcohol on breathing also accounts, in part, for the fact that if a person has excess alcohol before falling asleep at night, they can fall asleep faster but will wake up unrefreshed.

Blocked nose

Breathing through the nose is our normal way of breathing. If a person has a blocked nose because of previous trauma, allergic rhinitis, hay fever or upper respiratory tract infection, snoring and sleep apnoea are more likely to occur.

This is one of the reasons why there are commercially available devices that can be put either inside the nostril or outside (nasal strips) to try and improve nasal breathing. By and large, these devices have not been shown to be effective, but occasionally patients report improvement.

Hormonal problems

Patients with insufficient thyroid hormone (hypothyroidism) or an excess of growth hormone are at increased risk of snoring and sleep apnoea. People who suffer from diabetes are also more prone to experience sleep apnoea.

The frequency of sleep apnoea increases in women after the menopause, which suggests that female hormones may reduce the risk of snoring and obstructive sleep apnoea.

Smoking

Although less important than obesity and alcohol, smokers have chronic inflammation of the lining of the throat which can make apnoea more likely.

Male gender

Men are four times more likely to have sleep apnoea than women. This is probably due to hormonal influences, as gender differences tend to disappear after menopause. In children before puberty, the risk is the same between boys and girls.

There are other factors and other rare medical conditions

that can make sleep apnoea more likely. For example, people with a very small chin, children with cranio-facial abnormality and people with Marfan's syndrome[1] are more likely to have sleep apnoea.

What to do if you suspect obstructive sleep apnoea

Sleep apnoea is well known to medical practitioners and you should discuss your concerns with your family doctor. Depending on the situation, further investigation may be needed.

A simple home test called *oximetry* (Chapter 2) can be done as a screening test. The person's oxygen is monitored through a finger clip and up to eight hours of information can be stored in a computer chip. If a person is a snorer but does not stop breathing, the oxygen remains unchanged through the night with values above 90 per cent (see Chapter 2, Figure 11). However, if the person is stopping breathing, the oxygen level will fluctuate up and down, which is suggestive of sleep apnoea. The most comprehensive test available is the overnight sleep study described in Chapter 2.

Treatment of obstructive sleep apnoea

Weight reduction

For the large majority of patients with sleep apnoea, weight reduction is the most important treatment but also the most difficult to achieve. It is the only *cure* available; the other

---

1   Patients with Marfan's syndrome are tall and thin, with long arms and legs. They often have very loose joints. For example, they can bend their thumbs backwards down to their wrists.

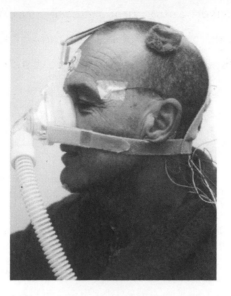

Figure 16   Nasal continuous positive airway pressure (CPAP)

forms of treatment improve *symptoms* but do not cure the condition.

Nasal continuous positive airway pressure (nCPAP)

A mask is attached to the nose while air is blown through a tube connected to a sophisticated compressor (Figure 16). This increases the pressure in the back of the throat, preventing it from collapsing by creating a pneumatic splint. It is a very effective treatment but cumbersome and impractical. About 25 per cent of patients cannot use it. It is, however, the treatment of choice for severe sleep apnoea (that is, stopping breathing more than thirty times an hour).

A variation of nasal CPAP is called *bi-level positive airway pressure*. With these devices the pressure increases when the person breathes in and decreases when the person breathes out which makes it easier to use.

Mandibular advancement devices (mouthguards)

These devices are oral appliances similar to the mouthguards used by patients who grind their teeth, and the ones used in sport. They are usually made of soft material, and the mould is taken with the lower jaw in a forward position. There are many different kinds of mouthguards available commercially, but the principle of action is the same. It is proposed that they modify the position of the lower jaw, together with the base of the tongue and the soft tissue structure of the throat. The forward and slightly downward positioning of the lower jaw may bring about an increase in space in the back of the throat, as well as altering the mechanical properties of the soft tissue of the palate.

Mouthguards are effective in about 70–80 per cent of patients who snore and are also indicated in mild sleep apnoea (stopping breathing less than thirty times an hour). They can also be tried in patients with severe sleep apnoea who cannot tolerate or do not want to use nasal CPAP.

The use of mouthguards can cause teeth discomfort in the morning and extra salivation. It is important that the bite is centred, otherwise temporo-mandibular pain (jaw pain) can result. Teeth need to be well maintained for a mouthguard to be applied.

Surgery to the palate

Surgery to the palate is called *uvulopalatopharyngoplasty* (Figure 17), often shortened to UPPP. It was initially thought that surgery could be a curative procedure for sleep apnoea. However, this is not the case and results suggest the following:

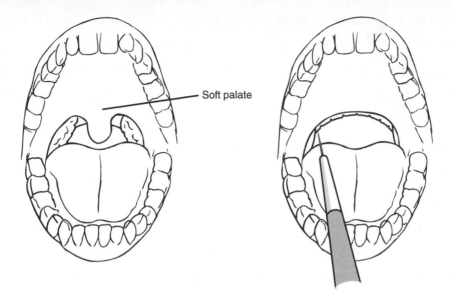

**Figure 17   Uvulopalatopharyngoplasty (UPPP), surgical
treatment of snoring**

- Surgery is not indicated in patients with severe sleep apnoea. In this setting the benefit is usually limited, with a recurrence of stopping breathing within a few months of the surgery.
- Surgery is an effective treatment for snoring and in some patients with mild sleep apnoea.
- Surgery to the palate does not bring about a permanent cure. This is to say that, as time passes, there is a risk of snoring recurring. This is particularly true if the person puts on weight.

There are potential complications due to surgery. The area that is operated on is involved with swallowing mechanisms, as well as with voice production. Although rare, after surgery some patients may have difficulty swallowing and the characteristics of the voice may change. This may be relevant in people who use their voice for professional reasons.

It should also be considered that, although the soft palate is the most common site of vibration causing snoring, in some people the site of vibration is the back of the tongue. In this situation, surgery to the palate will be ineffective. Currently, there is no certain way to identify the patients who have this problem.

Surgery to the palate can either be done with a scalpel or with a laser beam. Both procedures are painful, and the 'laser' treatment, when done in one session, is particularly painful. The laser treatment is a more recent technique and long-term consequences are not fully known.

Other surgical techniques can be applied to the mandible in an effort to bring it forward. These are performed in the United States but are not common in Australia.

✳ Upper airway resistance syndrome and central sleep apnoea

Two further conditions in which breathing is disturbed during sleep are upper airway resistance syndrome and central sleep apnoea.

Upper airway resistance syndrome is a condition half-way between pure snoring (noise making) and obstructive sleep apnoea. In upper airway resistance syndrome the patient does not stop breathing and therefore the oxygen level does not drop like it does with sleep apnoea. However, the body has to perform extra work to drive the air through the narrow passage of the throat during breathing. This extra effort causes disruption of sleep from a deep stage to a lighter stage. The person does not necessarily wake up completely, but their sleep is broken and often unrefreshing. The symptoms of upper airway resistance syndrome are the same as for obstructive sleep apnoea.

The term *sleep apnoea* usually refers to *obstructive* sleep apnoea, but often the word 'obstructive' is omitted. Collapse of the muscles at the level of the throat during sleep is the most common cause of sleep apnoea, accounting for 95 per cent of cases. However, there is another form of sleep apnoea called *central sleep apnoea* where the mechanism of stopping breathing is different. Central sleep apnoea is sometimes seen in children, often without causing any symptoms. It is also seen in patients with heart failure or who have previously suffered a stroke. In central sleep apnoea the person stops breathing because the breathing centre in the brain, located in close proximity to the sleep–wake centre, does not send information to the breathing muscles. The symptoms are similar to obstructive sleep apnoea, but treatment is more difficult and often not successful.

Ondine's curse is a rare form of central sleep apnoea seen in neonates and infants. In this condition the respiratory centre in the brain stem (see Figure 1 in Chapter 1) is not functioning well and causes apnoeas. The young patients stop breathing when asleep but *also* when awake. The condition can occur in adults following damage to some part of the brain. The name *Ondine's curse* is taken from a legend about a nymph, Ondine, who, having been abandoned by her husband, condemned him to having to remember to breathe in order to continue to live.

Treatment of upper airway resistance syndrome

The treatment of this condition is the same as for sleep apnoea. However, in upper airway resistance syndrome, weight reduction is paramount and usually effective.

Treatment of central sleep apnoea

Treatment is difficult because use of nasal CPAP is usually not effective. The problem in central sleep apnoea is not obstruction at the level of the palate. Instead, the breathing centre does not supply the appropriate information to the breathing muscles. Some beneficial effect is obtained by the use of a medication called theophylline, which was extensively used in the past for the treatment of asthma (Theodur™).

✳ Pregnancy, snoring and sleep apnoea

Snoring and sleep apnoea are less common in women than in men. However, during pregnancy important changes occur in a woman's body that may make snoring and sleep apnoea more likely. In particular, fluid retention (accumulation of fluid) may contribute to narrowing of the airways. Snoring is reported by 14 per cent of pregnant women, compared to 4 per cent of non-pregnant ones. In the third trimester it is more common, with 27 per cent of women reporting snoring. Snoring itself does not appear to increase the risks associated with delivery or to cause foetal distress. However, cases of obese women with sleep apnoea (snoring *and* stopping breathing) in whom pregnancy was complicated by foetal distress have been documented. In pre-eclampsia, a condition characterised by high blood pressure and marked fluid retention, congestion of the airways may precipitate disturbed breathing during sleep and result in a low oxygen level with potential increased risk for the foetus. An overnight sleep study can be performed safely in pregnancy and may help to clarify if sleep apnoea is present.

The treatment of these conditions in pregnancy is the same as in non-pregnant women.

✳ Other causes of 'choking' sensations during sleep

Although obstructive sleep apnoea is a common cause of waking up from sleep with choking sensations, the following conditions can also be causes of choking during sleep.

Gastric reflux (hiatus hernia)

This a very common complaint. Reflux is caused by fluid from the stomach coming back in the gullet and sometimes in the throat. Usually the person is aware of it because of a burning feeling in the chest (heartburn). However, one in four people with reflux do not have heartburn and therefore may not be aware of it. During sleep, when the muscles relax, a small amount of fluid can reach the throat and irritate the voice box and even spill into the trachea and bronchi. The person may wake up with a choking feeling. In sleep apnoea the sensation lasts only a second or two. In reflux the choking can last ten to twenty seconds or more and there is also prolonged coughing.

Avoidance of food and fluids in the two to three hours

before going to bed may help, together with medical treatment of reflux.

Panic attack, sleep laryngospasm and sleep choking syndrome

Many people are unaware that panic attacks can occur during sleep. The person wakes up with the sensation of not being able to *breathe in* (as opposed to asthma, where the difficulty is mostly to breathe out). There is also a feeling of anxiety, sometimes of impending doom and fright. As a spontaneous reaction the person tries to breathe harder. The harder they breathe, the more difficult it seems. The condition is frightening but not life-threatening. It can last a few minutes and then resolve itself. Treatment requires the person to become aware of this mechanism and then to try and breathe slowly. Explanation and reassurance is often all that is needed. If it happens frequently, benzodiazepine or other anti-anxiety medication can be very useful. People with this presentation are sometimes said to have *sleep laryngospam* or *sleep choking syndrome*.

4

Body jerks and restless limbs

- The majority of abnormal behaviours during sleep are not due to epilepsy.
- The cause of restless legs and periodic limb movement disorder is not known. They can fluctuate in severity.
- Sleep walking is very common up to fifteen years of age and usually does not require treatment.
- In nightmares the person recalls a frightening dream. In night terrors there is no dream recollection.
- In REM behaviour disorder the person acts out their dreams and can injure themself or their bed partner.
- Nocturnal epilepsy, and in particular frontal lobe epilepsy, can be difficult to recognise.

Regular change of position every twenty to thirty minutes is normal during sleep. Change in position is essential to avoid damage to the skin and muscles. People who are unconscious, drunk or suffering drug overdose and remain in the same position for hours can suffer injury with breakdown of skin and muscle, sometimes causing kidney failure and limb amputation.

However, other abnormal movements or complex behaviour may occur during sleep. They are known under the name of *parasomnias* and include:

- sleep starts (hypnic jerks);
- restless legs and periodic limb movement disorder;
- sleep talking;
- sleep walking;
- sleep drunkenness;
- sleep terrors;
- nightmares;
- REM sleep behaviour disorder;
- sleep epilepsy; and
- teeth grinding (bruxism).

✳ Sleep starts (hypnic jerks)

Sleep starts, or hypnic jerks, are sudden movements occurring *at sleep onset* and may be associated with a feeling of falling, imbalance or flowing. They are experienced by virtually everyone at some stage, and do not cause any harm or require treatment. They seem to be more common after exertion, emotional stress, and excess coffee or tea. Attention to these factors will reduce the frequency of sleep starts. If sleep starts are frequent and bothersome, a mild sedative at bedtime may be used on occasion.

✳ Restless legs and periodic limb movement disorder

Restless legs, sometimes called *Ekbom syndrome*, and periodic limb movement disorder are separate but closely related conditions. They are very common, being reported by 3 and 10 per cent of the general population, respectively.

Restless legs occurs equally in men and women. The typical complaint is of discomfort in the legs, mainly in the calves, but sometimes in the thighs. The sensation is described as crawling, or pins and needles, or cramping. The feeling is unpleasant, although not painful. Restless legs affects both legs and can occur during the day, but is more noticeable around bedtime. The discomfort is relieved by moving the legs or walking. The person often says that they are compelled to move their legs.

The majority of people with restless legs also have periodic limb movement disorder (PLMD) during sleep. However, patients with periodic limb movement disorder may not complain of restless leg during the day.

Limb movement refers to brief jerks of the ankles, knees, hips or arms which occur while the person is asleep and therefore unaware of it. The bed partner, however, is the one reporting the problem and complains of being 'kicked' all night. PLMD causes a lightening up of sleep. The person goes from deep sleep to light sleep each time a jerk occurs. Occasionally they can wake up completely for what appears to be 'no obvious reason'. If the jerks are frequent the person may complain of insomnia—of not being able to fall asleep or to remain asleep through the night. They wake up unrefreshed and feel tired during the day.

Periodic limb movements are different from sleep starts in that sleep starts occur as the person *is falling asleep* and often is aware of it. PLMD occurs *during sleep*. People with PLMD may complain of insomnia, difficulty initiating and maintaining sleep, daytime sleepiness, tiredness and chronic fatigue.

Causes and predisposing factors

It is unclear what causes restless legs and periodic limb movement disorder. Often they occur in families, which suggests a genetic influence. They appear to be more common with increasing age, even though often without untoward effects. They occur more commonly in iron deficiency, kidney failure and pregnancy. Certain medications used for depression, tricyclic antidepressants (amitriptyline, doxepin and imipramine) can worsen or trigger periodic limb movements. Withdrawal from benzodiazepines (diazepam, temazepam, oxazepam and nitrazepam) can also make limb movement worse.

In the condition called *fibromyalgia* or *fibrositis*, periodic limb movements are said to be more common. This condition is a variant of chronic fatigue syndrome, with frequent muscle and joint aches and unrefreshed sleep.

Other reasons for 'aching' and 'jerking' legs

There are many reasons for leg discomfort, including varicose veins, poor circulation, damage to the nerves (neuropathy), chronic lumbar spine problems and vein clots. People who are on fluid tablets, which often lower the body content of salt, often complain of aching legs.

How to confirm restless legs and PLMD

The history is usually sufficient provided that the other possibilities mentioned in the previous paragraph are excluded. However, if there are any doubts, an overnight sleep study will help confirm the diagnosis (Figure 18).

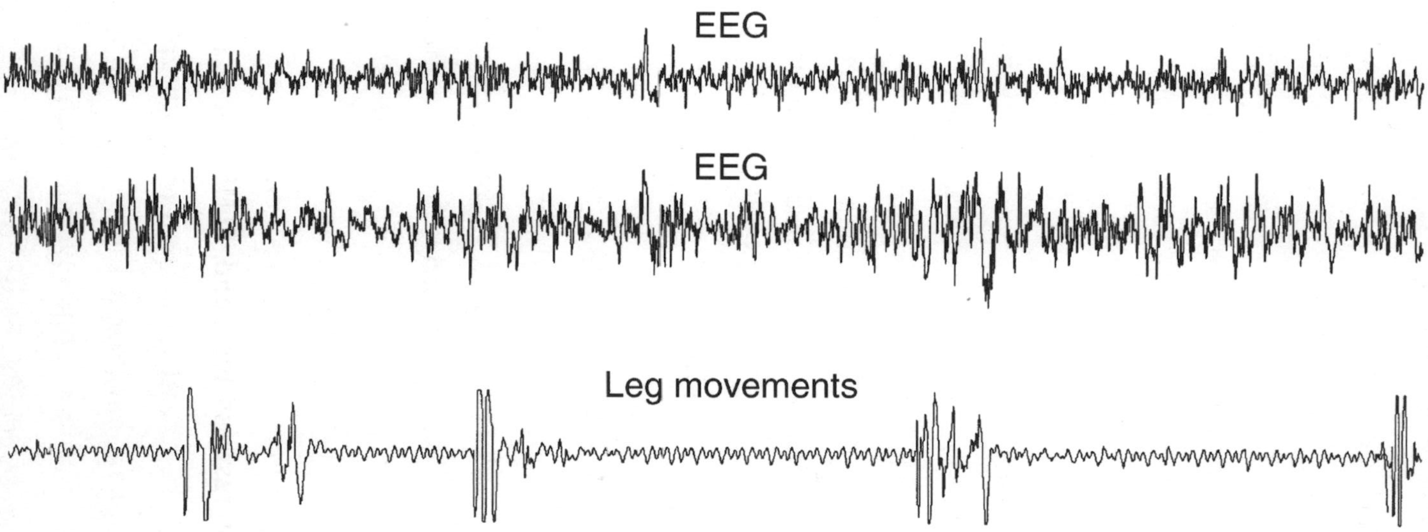

EEG

EEG

Leg movements

Figure 18 Five leg movements were recorded over one minute during sleep using a sensor positioned over the patient's shin

Treatment

The severity of restless legs and PLMD varies from being an occasional nuisance to being a daily debilitating condition. The first approach is to avoid, if possible, trigger factors—that is, correction of iron deficiency and avoidance of medications such as tricyclic antidepressants and excessive caffeinated beverages. When needed, two groups of medications are useful in these conditions: opioids (morphine and codeine) and benzodiazepines. Morphine is probably the most effective medication, but, like codeine, it can cause constipation, problems with voiding, and nausea and may be avoided by people because of the risk of 'addiction'. The concern about addiction, which also involves benzodiazepines, is overstated, particularly considering that the medication is taken for a specific medical condition and under medical supervision.

Our practice is to start the person with short-acting benzodiazepines such as temazepam (one or two tablets—10–20 milligrams—at bedtime). A similar medication that people may have been started on in the past, called Rivotril™, is not available at present because of Medicare restrictions. Codeine (30–60 milligrams at bedtime) or morphine (up to 40–50 milligrams) is effective in suppressing the symptoms.

We usually recommend that the medication is used daily for two or three weeks; after that, it can be reduced to every second day or simply 'when needed'. In severe conditions the medication has to be taken daily for a long time. Although treatment is usually given at night, some people with restless legs may need to take a dose in the morning as well.

It should be stressed that the symptoms can fluctuate spontaneously over time. This is to say that the person can improve with no treatment.

Quinate tablets are frequently used by people with symptoms of cramps in the calves with some documented effect. Natural products such as ginseng and ginkgo-biloba are often used, but are not useful in our experience.

The use of anti-Parkinson's disease medications such as Sinemet™ or Madopar™ is sometimes advocated. We have not found these medications consistently useful and they are difficult to manage.

❋ Sleep talking

Sleep talking is a common event during sleep. It can occur during both REM and non-REM sleep. It is often associated with other activities such as sleep walking. The person has no recollection of the words, which at times are incomprehensible.

There is often a family history of sleep talking. Contrary to common belief, there is no relation with anxiety or depression. No treatment is necessary.

❋ Sleep walking

Sleep walking refers to both simple and complex behaviour during sleep. The sleep walker can simply sit up in bed and move their arms and head around, either with their eyes open or closed, or they can get out of bed and perform complex and prolonged tasks. They are difficult to arouse and, when awakened, can be disoriented for a minute or two. The person has no recollection of the event. Sleep talking is often present as well.

Sleep walking has attracted vast interest spanning from literature and folklore to the legal system. The belief that sleep walkers can perform risky tasks safely, such as walking along a balcony railing or a tightrope, is simply not true. However, severe injuries do occur when people go through glass doors, fall out of windows, or leave a gas outlet opened.

Of media interest are situations where a crime is committed in an alleged sleep-walking state. Although open to debate, it is recognised that complex behaviour can occur during sleep walking, including criminal action. The legal implications are important because, in this circumstance, the offender may be considered not responsible for their actions because of lack of consciousness.

Sleep walking is mostly a condition of childhood, with onset between four and six years of age and remission by the teenage years. However, it may persist into adulthood. When sleep walking *starts* in adulthood without having been present as a child, other possibilities need to be considered. Specifically, a form of epilepsy called *complex partial seizures* needs to be excluded. In this group of people, psychological disturbances such as anxiety, depression or manic personality are said to be common, but evidence for these claims is only anecdotal.

Sleep walking occurs during a part of sleep called *slow wave sleep* (non-REM sleep) and is more common during the first part of the night. The cause of sleep walking is not known. Like sleep talking, it can run in families, with increased risk if both parents have suffered from it. Physical tiredness and sleep deprivation can trigger sleep walking.

Conditions similar to sleep walking

Complex activities during sleep may be due to other sleep disorders such as epilepsy, REM behaviour disorder, night terrors and sleep drunkenness, as described below.

Treatment is rarely needed except when people put themselves or others at risk. Reassurance and avoiding injury is often all that is needed. However, if the behaviour continues and is dangerous, short-acting benzodiazepines such as temazepam, and tricyclic antidepressants such as imipramine, can be used on a 'when needed' basis.

✳ Sleep drunkenness

Sleep drunkenness is common in children and can occur in adults. It is a state of partial wakefulness where the person is 'half asleep and half awake'. When brain activity is monitored, it shows recurrent microsleep (a repetition of brief periods of wakefulness followed by brief periods of sleep). The person appears confused and disoriented. They may be able to respond to questions and commands. There is no recollection of the events when the person wakes in the morning. In children, sleep drunkenness is common if the child is woken up forcefully from deep sleep in the middle of the night. In adults, it is seen in patients with sleep apnoea and those in states of increased sleepiness, such as persons with chronic sleep deprivation and narcolepsy. Reassurance that the condition is benign is usually sufficient.

✳ Sleep terrors

Sleep terrors also occur during the period of slow wave sleep and often coexist with sleep walking. The condition is more common in toddlers and young children and tends to resolve spontaneously. Sleep terrors are of sudden onset. The child sits up in bed, often with screaming and vocalisations that are usually not comprehensible. They may leave the bed or fight if someone tries to console or restrain them. The episode settles spontaneously and the person goes back to sleep.

If the child is awakened, they may be disoriented and have no recollection of the event or of any dreaming. Bed wetting can occur during these episodes.

Like sleep walking, there may be a family history of sleep terrors. Tiredness, fever and prior sleep deprivation can be a trigger.

In childhood, sleep terrors are not suggestive of psychopathology, but onset in adolescence and adulthood may be associated with psychiatric illnesses.

Apart from reassurance and avoidance of injury, which may occur if the child runs out of bed, no other treatment is needed except in exceptional circumstances where the use of benzodiazepine or imipramine can be considered.

✳ Nightmares

Nightmares are described here because they are often confused with night terrors and REM behaviour disorder. Nightmares are different from sleep terrors, because they usually occur during REM sleep and are frightening dreams that cause anxiety. Unlike sleep terrors, the person has recollection of nightmares. They can start at any age.

Prolonged stressful situations can result in increased frequency of nightmares. Over 50 per cent of patients with post-traumatic stress disorder (PTSD) report nightmares once a month, compared to 24 per cent of young students who report them once a year. Medications for high blood pressure and Parkinson's disease, such as beta-blockers and L-dopa, can increase the risk of nightmares. They occur in a majority of people at some stage in life.

Treatment may be needed if they are frequent. Simple reassurance can be sufficient. Counselling regarding ongoing stress, or specific psychiatric treatment, may be needed. Medications that suppress rapid eye movement are useful and include benzodiazepine and tricyclic antidepressants. Treatment will be continued for a few weeks and then tapered off slowly.

✳ REM sleep behaviour disorder

This is a condition usually seen in middle-aged and elderly men and rarely in women or young people. It results from 'acting out of dreams'.

In REM sleep behaviour disorder, patients can make violent movements during sleep which can lead to injury to themselves or their bed partner. The patient can punch, kick, leap out of bed, or even run from the bed in an attempted enactment of dreams. This behaviour during sleep can occur occasionally or up to three or four times a night on consecutive nights.

In the majority of cases, there is no obvious reason for it. Occasionally, it can occur following withdrawal from alcohol, sedatives or antidepressant medication. There is an association between REM behaviour disorders and neurological abnormalities such as Parkinson's disease, dementia and previous stroke.

Treatment, when needed, involves the use of medication that suppresses rapid eye movement. A medication called clonazepam (Rivotril™), was used in the past until it was made unavailable due to Medicare restrictions, and was usually effective. Other benzodiazepines can also be used.

REM behaviour disorder can be confused with nocturnal epilepsy and, in particular, with frontal lobe epilepsy (see below).

❊ Sleep epilepsy

Some forms of epilepsy only occur during sleep. The typical form of epilepsy, where the person initially becomes rigid and stiff with grunting noises followed by jerky movements, is easily recognisable as epilepsy if witnessed. The person can wet themself, bite their tongue or lips, and experience a prolonged period of drowsiness after the seizure is finished. In a form of epilepsy called *temporal lobe epilepsy*, or *psychomotor epilepsy*, the person's behaviour can be difficult to distinguish from sleep walking. In epilepsy, however, movements are often repetitive. The person is less likely to go back to bed and resume sleep, as happens in sleep walking.

The use of special tests such as an EEG (electroencephalogram) and a sleep study with videotaping can help to distinguish between the forms of abnormal behaviour during sleep.

One particular form of epilepsy, called *frontal lobe epilepsy*, is worth mentioning. It occurs during sleep and is often not recognised, or is mistaken for other movement disorders. Frontal lobe epilepsy is genetic, and there may be a family history of it, unless it has not previously been recognised. It starts in childhood or adolescence. It varies in severity from simple repeated stroking of the nose or waving of the arms, to strong, rhythmic jerks that can shake the bed. The activity can last from three to four seconds to more than a minute. Epileptic activity in the brain is recorded only during an attack, but not between seizures. Therefore, an EEG recorded during the day may appear normal. This makes the diagnosis difficult.

The characteristic of frontal lobe epilepsy is that the motor activity (stroking of the nose or of the ear, or jerky movements) is always the same, night by night. Observation by the bed partner or parents of the repetitive nature of the movement should raise suspicion. Frontal lobe epilepsy tends to occur at any time during the night, while sleep walking is more common in the first part of the night. Also, the abnormal behaviour due to frontal lobe epilepsy is frequent, occurring on many nights each week, contrary to the other parasomnias which are less frequent.

Treatment is with a medication called carbamazepine (Tegretol™) or clonazepam (Rivotril™) taken at night. Rivotril™ use is allowed for this condition under Medicare.

✳ Teeth grinding (bruxism)

Teeth grinding, or bruxism, is common both in men and women. It may be an occasional complaint, occurring only during periods of stress, or a regular event. It often starts in childhood and may be diagnosed by a dentist who notices damage to the teeth due to mechanical attrition. The noise produced by teeth grinding can be loud and unpleasant. The person themself may not be aware, or may complain of a sore jaw in the morning. Bruxism is more common in certain families. An important and remediable cause of teeth grinding is poor dental occlusion. If dental contacts and alignment are abnormal, this can trigger spasms in the jaw muscles and result in bruxism. In this case, dental treatment, including orthodontics, is needed.

It is well documented that a high level of stress predisposes to teeth grinding and that it is more common in anxious people. High alcohol intake (four or more standard drinks) is said to increase bruxism.

Treatment is not needed if the condition is rare. Proper dental care, with optimisation of occlusion, and sometimes a mouthguard, are usually effective. If this treatment fails or is not possible, benzodiazepines are useful—in particular, in anxious people and when stress is present.

5

Insomnia

- Insomnia is a symptom, not a disease.
- Insomnia is a symptom of daytime malfunction and not just a nighttime problem.
- A careful history of medications used, medical problems, and personal/ interpersonal (family, job) problems needs to be taken.
- Be aware of the psychophysiological mechanism which perpetuates insomnia.
- Treatment needs to address the causes of insomnia, rather than insomnia itself.

People complaining of insomnia are unsatisfied with the quality of their sleep. Two points are paramount in understanding insomnia:

- Insomnia is a symptom, not a disease.
- Insomnia is a symptom of daytime dysfunction as well as of poor nighttime sleep.

A person presenting with insomnia complains of one or more of the following:

- difficulty initiating sleep;
- difficulty maintaining sleep;
- early-morning arousal; and/or
- fatigue and tiredness, with mood changes during the day.

It is the *quality* and *perception* of the time spent asleep, more than the amount of hours that are important in insomnia.

It cannot be overemphasised that *insomnia is a symptom and not a disease*. This is to say that having insomnia is like having a headache. Some people *never* have headaches; others may have the occasional headache lasting a day or two. However, people with migraine may have headaches every month, and some unfortunate ones may have them every day and need continual medication to reduce their suffering. A headache can be a symptom of a sinister disease such as meningitis or even of a brain tumour. It is unclear why some people develop tension headaches during stressful situations and others don't, but it is thought that it may have to do with 'personality'.

Similarly, insomnia can be a complaint limited to a few days or a few weeks, due to a stressful event. A relationship problem, a financial crisis, an exam or a death in the family are examples of situations when the level of anxiety rises and may result in difficulty initiating and maintaining sleep. The effect varies from one person to another, but it can affect everyone. It should be stressed that in this condition the person sleeps poorly at night, as well as functioning poorly during the day. Someone who is grieving the loss of someone dear may not only have difficulty sleeping but is also likely to be affected in their job, as well as in their relationships with others, during the day.

From a practical point of view, insomnia in this situation is regarded as a normal reaction of the body in difficult circumstances. It is referred to as *transient* or *short-term insomnia*. The person is usually aware that the insomnia is triggered by an ongoing problem and rarely seeks medical advice. No specific intervention is needed, but on occasion hypnotic medications (medications that promote sleep) are required for a brief period of time. Sleep disorders centres do not usually see people with transient or short-term insomnia; rather, they assess patients with chronic or persistent insomnia.

❊ Chronic insomnia

By convention, chronic insomnia is said to be present if symptoms persist for more than six months. In the majority of people we see, insomnia has been present for many years—often, for as long as they can remember. Because insomnia is a symptom and not a disease, the first question to consider is: 'In this person, what is chronic insomnia a symptom of?'

However, before considering this question, two very important points need to be made.

- Sleep is different in different people.
- Psychophysiological insomnia is a variety of insomnia in which this mechanism is the predominant (only) cause of the symptoms.

Sleep is different in different people

This point was stressed in Chapter 1 and is applicable to all sleep disorders, including insomnia. Chronic insomnia may be more common in women than in men, and with increasing age. Genetic influences are also at work in insomnia, to varying degrees. This is exemplified in the condition called *idiopathic insomnia*, or *childhood onset insomnia*.

This type of insomnia starts in very early childhood and tends to persist through life. There is often a family history of it. Both the person themself and their family recall difficulty in falling asleep and staying asleep going back to a very early age. Although no specific abnormalities are found, it is presumed that there is a dysfunction of the wake–sleep system that is responsible for the insomnia. People with childhood onset insomnia do not have psychological or psychiatric abnormality; however, when the condition is severe it may result in social disruption due to poor ability to perform, chronic tiredness, inability to concentrate and memory disturbances.

Psychophysiological mechanism

Psychophysiological mechanism operates in almost all forms of chronic insomnia, increasing the severity of the symptoms and maintaining insomnia over time. In some people, the insomnia started many years previously with what appears to have been a transient problem. The person recalls a period of high stress, for any reason, which caused a high level of anxiety and resulted in difficulty initiating and maintaining sleep. However, the symptoms, instead of resolving after a few weeks, persisted, reinforcing themselves as time passed. The reason why this happens can be explained by two factors:

- *Personality*. Some people tend to be light sleepers to begin with and react to stressful situations with high levels of tension.
- *Insomnia reinforcing itself*. The insomnia 'feeds' on itself. Because sleep quality fails to improve over time, the person

becomes progressively more focused on the need to 'get a good night's sleep at last'. However, as bedtime approaches, the harder they try to get a good night's sleep, the more their level of anxiety rises. This results in further deterioration of their ability to initiate and maintain sleep. The person then tries to help sleep with activities such as relaxation techniques, reading or listening to music in bed, or watching television. All of these measures initially tend to help a little. However, they become less effective over time. The result is that, the bed and bedroom, instead of being the place where the person rests, becomes an anxiety-producing environment. As bedtime approaches, the person becomes progressively more concerned that they won't sleep again, and will feel so tired the next day that they won't be able to carry out their duties. In simple terms, the person feels that they *have lost control over their sleep*. The result is a feeling of chronic tiredness, an inability to perform properly during the day and, often, a chronically depressed mood.

So, keeping in mind that quality of sleep varies among individuals and that psychophysiological mechanisms are often present, the first question to answer is: What causes insomnia?

❊ Causes of insomnia

Medical problems

Any chronic medical condition that interrupts sleep may cause chronic insomnia. For example, asthma gets worse at night and a poorly controlled asthmatic may experience coughing and wheezing during sleep, often causing recurrent arousals (waking up). People with poorly controlled heart failure tend to wake up with shortness of breath many times during the night. Patients with chronic back pain due to osteoporosis, osteoarthritis or rheumatoid arthritis may have poor sleep if pain is not controlled. Thyrotoxicosis, an increase in thyroid hormones, tends to cause insomnia. These are only a few examples. Even in this group of patients a psycho-physiological mechanism can set in, making the symptoms worse.

Treatment needs to be directed at improving the medical condition in question. This is one reason why people with insomnia should have a thorough medical assessment.

Menopause and female hormones

A subgroup of women can develop poor sleep quality, with difficulty maintaining sleep, at the time of the menopause. This appears to be related to a decrease in the level of female hormones. Oestrogen replacement has shown improvement in sleep quality, with shorter time to fall asleep, more REM sleep, and less wakefulness after sleep onset. Not all studies support this view. It has been argued that oestrogen improves perception of sleep by improving the sense of physical and psychological well-being, rather than by direct effect on sleep. In clinical practice it seems that some women's sleep patterns improve on hormone replacement, while others seem not to benefit. Unless there is a specific contraindication to use oestrogens, a trial of treatment is warranted if sleep difficulties start at the time of menopause.

Other 'sleep' disorders

Any other sleep disorder can present with difficulty initiating and maintaining sleep. It is common for people with sleep apnoea (see Chapter 3) to wake up recurrently through the night complaining of difficulty maintaining sleep.

People with periodic limb movement disorder (see Chapter 4) can complain of difficulty initiating sleep. Perhaps the most important group of sleep disorders that present complaining of insomnia and are often undiagnosed are *sleep timing disorders* such as advanced sleep phase syndrome and delayed sleep phase syndrome (see later in this chapter). For example, in delayed sleep phase syndrome, the use of medication, relaxation techniques and other strategies is usually unsuccessful. In insomnia due to sleep timing disorder, light therapy and, possibly, melatonin are useful treatments. When insomnia is a symptom of sleep disorders, an overnight sleep study helps to clarify the diagnosis.

Psychiatric illness

People with psychiatric illness are unwell during the day and sleep poorly at night. Insomnia is common in people with manic depressive illness and those with anxiety disorder. It should be stressed that the word 'depression' is used for both reactive depression and primary depression, even though the two conditions are somewhat different. *Reactive depression* is common and refers to depressed mood as a consequence of poor general health, or difficult or prolonged personal or social situations. A person who has been made redundant and cannot find a job may go through a period of depressed mood and disturbed sleep. If this state of affairs continues long enough, not only will the person be emotionally depressed, but, not being able to sleep and rest, will also become physically unwell. The use of antidepressants is of little value, both for the depressed mood as well as for the insomnia. This person needs counselling and help in readjusting to his or her social situation. This is obviously much harder work than just taking tablets at nighttime. In *primary depression*, the depressed mood is a problem in itself and not a reaction to another problem. Insomnia in this setting requires psychiatric evaluation and treatment, and often the prolonged use of medication.

One particular form of depression, called *seasonal affective disorder* (SAD), is worth mentioning because of the associated sleep problem. SAD is more often reported in autumn and winter than in summer, and is more common in women. The person has difficulty falling asleep in a fashion similar to delayed sleep phase syndrome (see later in this chapter). They feel unrefreshed in the morning and lethargic during the day. It is felt that lack of sufficient exposure to light, due to increased indoor activity in the winter months, is a contributing factor. Seasonal affective disorder is more common in countries furthest away from the equator where daylight is very reduced in winter. The use of light therapy in the morning is an effective treatment (see later in this chapter).

Psychophysiological insomnia

As mentioned previously, psychophysiological mechanisms are likely to contribute to chronic insomnia symptoms in *all* cases, but it is a common, perhaps *the* most common, cause of chronic insomnia in its own right.

Although a trigger event is often present in psychophysiological insomnia, it is often forgotten, because usually the symptoms have been present for a long time. Sometimes, the person has been able to cope with the events in the past by forgetting them. In this situation an accurate history is needed.

The following two examples will clarify this issue further.

A 61-year-old man had experienced difficulty initiating and maintaining sleep for more than twenty years. Twelve months prior to being seen, he was diagnosed with lymphoma (cancer of the blood cells, which carries a 50 per cent risk of dying). He had undergone chemotherapy (drug treatment) for six months, with few side-effects and a good response (apparent cure). Over the last twelve months, his symptoms of insomnia had worsened, but he admitted that the problem had been present since his early forties. He was not able to volunteer any reason for it, or any particular trigger for it. However, after being asked if anything important had happened twenty years before in his personal or work life, he made a connection between the onset of insomnia and the death of his son at age seventeen. To use his own words, his son 'was such a good boy that I decided to buy him a car when he turned seventeen'. Unfortunately, a few days later, driving back home at night, his son hit a pole on the side of the road and died. The patient admitted that he had never completely recovered from his son's death. Even though at a rational level he may have come to terms with the death of his son, the emotional load associated with it, and the sense of guilt about having bought the car, had been a persistent thorn in his side. This was exacerbated by the fact that he had not gone through a full grieving process. He was on sleeping tablets for the first two years, and then on and off them after that, but he admitted that they made no difference to his sleep. Twenty years later, at the age of 61, when he had planned to retire and go travelling around Australia, as many Australians do, he was diagnosed with lymphoma. This had exacerbated his symptoms. Further use of sleeping tablets and antidepressants had made no difference to his insomnia.

For this man, understanding how his insomnia started, and confronting the negative feelings associated with the death of his son, were important starting points for treatment. The process was time-consuming and uncomfortable, but important, particularly when the only coping mechanism he had had was to try and forget the tragic event. Confronting and openly admitting his fear and anxiety after the diagnosis of lymphoma, and the potential threat of its recurrence, were also essential elements in his treatment. This awareness process was not only useful in improving his nighttime symptoms, but also had a positive effect on his ability to look ahead and plan for the future.

Sometimes a person may have problems relevant to their insomnia that cannot be resolved or changed. However, the process of fully evaluating them is often beneficial and sufficient treatment. In the case of the man in the example above, no counselling could change the fact of the death of his son.

It is also obvious that no tablet—be it Prozac™, Aropax™, Zoloft™ or Prothiaden™—can substitute for the above process. It would be convenient to be able to solve the problem with a tablet, but it doesn't work and may actually make things worse. In fact, it reinforces the idea that the insomnia is the reason why the person is unwell, when actually it is only one of the symptoms of a more complex situation.

This next example is also worth considering.

A 36-year-old woman was referred 'urgently' because of insomnia. The family doctor explained that the woman could not sleep at all, various medications had proved unhelpful, and she was becoming desperate.

She was a married professional working part-time, with three young children. She was healthy otherwise. The husband was a manager in a large firm, and they had just moved to town within the last twelve months.

The interview started with an open question: 'What is the problem as you see it?' She replied that in the last twelve months she had had difficulty falling asleep. She would wake up regularly in the middle of the night and stay awake, sometimes for hours. She had now got to the point where, unless she could get a good night's sleep, she felt she couldn't go on any longer. She had tried different sleeping tablets, including antidepressants, but to no avail. In fact, some of the medications made her feel worse during the day.

Consistent with the view that 'sleep disorders' are disorders of daytime as well as nighttime function, we started the patient's history from wake-up time. She said that she gets up at 6.30 a.m. to prepare her children and drive them to school. She then goes to work (twenty hours a week). She also attends a postgraduate course at the university two evenings a week.

After school she takes the children to swimming, Little Athletics and basketball three times a week and on Saturday morning. Then she has the housekeeping and shopping to do, along with her university work.

The husband, as a manager, leaves at 7 a.m. and returns home at 7 p.m.

A few observations can be made at this point. The patient had made some important decisions, such as working part-time in order to look after the family. Her work and career opportunities were subordinated to her husband's career. This was a conscious decision and one she did not regret.

The next question was: 'Do you have any time for *yourself*, for the things that *you* would like to do?' This was obviously a critical point, as the patient became visibly upset. She had moved to a new town with no family support around her. She had no one to leave the children with, even for a few hours. She attended to the needs of all the other family members, at the expense of her own needs, including her need to rest. She admitted to having a good relationship with her husband, who, however, seemed insensitive to her feeling unwell. His reaction was that he worked long hours too, but that he didn't complain about being tired.

In this case, the complaint of insomnia was a symptom of both physical and mental overwork and chronic sleep deprivation. The history, and a few simple investigations, excluded any other medical or psychiatric problem. Other sleep disorders were considered unlikely, but an overnight sleep study was undertaken. The patient slept well and the recording showed normal sleep quality as well as sleep structure. It is a common finding in psychophysiological insomnia that the person has a good night's sleep away from their usual environment.

Treatment was aimed at first acknowledging what the real issues were—in this patient's case, daytime was more important than nighttime.

Therefore, modification of daytime function was needed. Perhaps some home duties had to be delegated to a housekeeper and/or the children had to reduce their amount of after-school activity. Perhaps a babysitter could be employed for a few hours to give the woman and her husband some time on their own.

These are only two of many possible situations where insomnia is a symptom, and not the cause, of feeling unwell.

Sleep timing disorders

Within the group of timing disorders the most common are shift work, delayed sleep phase syndrome and advanced sleep phase syndrome. Shift work is considered in Chapter 6, but the other two conditions are dealt with here because patients with delayed and advanced phase syndrome present complaining of insomnia.

In timing disorders, sleep itself is normal, but the times when sleep starts and finishes are out of phase. The majority of people fall asleep between 8.30 p.m. and midnight. One group preferentially falls asleep between 8.30 and 10.30 p.m. ('larks'), and at 6.30–7 a.m. they are up and about without delay and ready to go. The second group ('owls') tends to fall asleep between 10.30 p.m. and midnight and would preferentially keep sleeping until 7.30–8 a.m. or later.

The importance of timing disorders is that patients present to their general practitioner complaining of insomnia. They report not being able to fall asleep or maintain sleep, or they wake too early and cannot go back to sleep. Sleeping tablets are not effective in these conditions and specific treatment is needed.

Delayed sleep phase syndrome

In this condition the person cannot fall asleep until after midnight, sometimes not until 2–3 a.m. In the morning they sleep until 10–11 a.m. This 'out-of-phase' situation, where sleep onset is delayed compared to the usual timing, may not be a problem if it suits the person's lifestyle. However, it usually becomes a problem because the person tries to fall asleep at the 'usual time'. For example, if someone with delayed sleep phase syndrome goes to bed at 10 p.m. they may toss and turn for two to three hours, becoming progressively more anxious and angry with themself because of their inability to fall asleep. The usual remedies—reading, listening to music or relaxation tapes, autohypnosis and sleeping tablets—don't work. At best, even when exhausted, the person may fall asleep for thirty to sixty minutes and then find themself wide awake until 1–2 a.m. when finally the body is ready to fall asleep.

In the morning, as the majority of us need to get up between 6–7 a.m. to go to work or school, such a person has only been able to get four to five hours of sleep at best. They become progressively sleep deprived, chronically tired, both mentally and physically, and their function during the day deteriorates. The following night they feel very tired and would like to have an early night to catch up with sleep. But once again, they are unable to fall asleep until the early hours of the morning. This situation can continue in a vicious circle, with an element of psychophysiological insomnia also setting in.

Causes of delayed sleep phase syndrome

A typical situation where delayed sleep phase syndrome develops is in university students during their examinations, when they keep working until 1–2 a.m. for two to three weeks. When the exam period is eventually over, some students find it difficult to go back to a normal bedtime routine. Any situation where a person delays sleep time until the early hours of the morning for weeks, or sometimes months, may cause the onset of a delayed sleep phase syndrome. Although delayed sleep phase syndrome can set in at any age, it starts more commonly in teenagers and young adults (perhaps because of social factors). A family tendency seems also to predispose to it.

Treatment

Treatment involves the following three strategies:

- restriction of time in bed;
- 'light' therapy in the morning; and
- melatonin.

The patient should try and go to bed late, preferably around midnight. Irrespective of the amount of sleep achieved, they should get up at 6–6.30 a.m. and expose themself to bright light for half an hour or an hour. Natural light (outdoors) is preferable and the easiest way in summer. In winter, a light box may be used instead. Artificial light needs to be at least 2500 *lux*, which is the equivalent of a bright x-ray box. (One *lux* is the amount of light emitted by a candle at a distance of one metre.)

The principle behind using bright light is to 'trick the body' into thinking it is later in the day, and this may result in anticipating the clock. An advancement of one to two hours can be achieved by the exposure to bright light in the morning for one to two hours. The more powerful the light, the greater the effect. Although the distance and positioning of the light source (directly in front, sideways or ceiling reflected light) are subject to some debate, it seems unnecessary to stare directly at the light to obtain the benefit. Going for a walk, or having breakfast on the verandah or in the garden, is ideal as it provides between 3000 and 10 000 *lux*, depending on whether the day is clear or cloudy. If this is not possible or practical, such as in winter, a light box is usually effective. Commercial light boxes are available in certain countries (see Appendix 2), but not currently in Australia. A light box can be built by a qualified electrician using a fluorescent light source in the range of 200 to 300 watts. A plastic diffuser should be used to filter ultraviolet light, which is harmful to the eyes.

More recently, melatonin has been suggested as a potential treatment. Melatonin is used early in the evening, at 8–9 p.m., and may help in advancing the body clock.

The combination of restriction of time in bed, bright light in the morning and melatonin in the evening may have an additive effect.

Advanced sleep phase syndrome

In this condition the person is ready to sleep by 7–8 p.m., then at 1–2 a.m. they wake up and are unable to go back to sleep.

These people often take a nap in the early afternoon as they have been awake since the early morning.

Advanced sleep phase syndrome is typically seen in elderly people whose sleep is already reduced because of age and often more fragmented.

Treatment

Often treatment is not needed if the phase shift is not interfering with daily function. The use of bright light in the evening, at 6–7 p.m. for up to an hour may help delay bedtime for a few hours. The use of melatonin in the morning is also advocated in this situation. It should be noted again that sleeping tablets are neither useful nor successful in 'out-of-phase' disorders.

❋ How is chronic insomnia investigated?

From what we have said so far, we can summarise as follows:

- Insomnia is a symptom, not a disease (with the exception, perhaps, of childhood onset insomnia).
- What happened during the day is as important in understanding insomnia as what happens at night.
- It is important to exclude medical conditions, which may be a cause of difficulty initiating and maintaining sleep.
- Many medications used for other medical conditions can cause insomnia. Notably the new group of antidepressants (Prozac™, Aropax™ and the like) can cause insomnia.
- Tea or coffee can cause insomnia in some people.

Psychiatric opinion

Sometimes a psychiatric interview can be useful. However, the suggestion of seeing a psychiatrist is usually ill-received. Seeing a psychiatrist has a bad connotation, because of the preconceived idea that psychiatrists see 'mad' people or that they may imply that the symptoms are 'only in your mind' and not real. However, a psychiatrist is only a professional with a specific interest and expertise in assessing the emotional aspects of the self, and this can be very useful. It may also reveal that the insomnia is a symptom of a primary psychiatric illness (for example, manic depression [now called bipolar disorder], anxiety disorder or schizophrenia) and that specific treatment is needed.

Sleep study

Many sleep disorders can present with difficulty initiating and maintaining sleep. Observing the person's sleep and recording their brain waves can sometimes be useful. In particular, sleep timing disorders often present with symptoms of insomnia.

Another interesting condition observed during sleep recording is *sleep misperception*. This is the situation where the person reports not being able to sleep for days at a time or for only an hour or so each night. They also often report not taking naps through the day. Although there are reports of people sleeping for only a few hours a night for many years, this is extremely rare. Patients with sleep misperception, following an overnight sleep study, report having slept for only a few minutes even when their brain wave activity shows six or seven hours of sleep. This is to say that the person actually slept for longer than they perceived. It is unclear why there is a difference between what is recorded and what the person feels. Perhaps our current understanding of sleep is not sophisticated enough to explain this finding. Treatment of sleep misperception is difficult, and medications are usually ineffective.

Sleep diary

A sleep diary is a useful way to assess what happens at night and how sleep patterns may change over time. (An example of the sleep diary we use appears as Figure 8 in Chapter 2.) Sleep diaries are also used when a technique called *restriction of time in bed* is undertaken (see below).

❋ Treatment of chronic insomnia

From what we have said so far, it can be deduced that treatment will depend on the underlying problem. Specific treatments are needed if a medical or psychiatric disease is present. The same applies if sleep disorders such as sleep apnoea, leg movement or sleep timing disorders are the cause of the problem.

When psychophysiological insomnia is the main issue the following treatments may be used.

Keeping a sleep diary

Keeping a sleep diary for a week or two gives the person a better understanding of their sleep and involves them directly in management of their treatment.

Reviewing the sleep–wake routine

Because insomnia has often been present for a long time, the person may have developed behaviour that affects sleep in an unfavourable manner. For instance, watching television in bed, or listening to relaxation tapes or to the radio, is not advisable. Drinking large amounts of tea or coffee during the day or alcohol to excess at night is best avoided. The same applies to daytime napping. Although taking a nap in the afternoon is quite appropriate, it is best avoided if insomnia is present. (See the suggestions for better sleep in the box on the following page.)

Maintaining a regular sleep time and wake-up time

Going to bed one night at 9 p.m. and the next night at midnight should be discouraged. When there is a sleep timing problem, a technique called *restriction of time in bed* can be useful. The following is an example.

A patient keeps a sleep diary for about ten days, which shows that on average he goes to bed at 11 p.m., takes about an hour to fall asleep, wakes up once during the night and is awake for an hour. He then falls asleep again and gets up at 7 a.m. This means that he is in bed for eight hours, but in effect he sleeps for only six out of those hours.

We then decide to restrict the time allowed in bed to six hours. The patient will go to bed at midnight and get up by the clock at 6 a.m. He is also not allowed to take any naps through the day. In doing so, he becomes somewhat sleep deprived, and when he hits the pillow at midnight sleep starts fairly quickly and tends to be more solid through the night. After a week or so, once this routine is consolidated, then either bedtime or get-up time is changed. For example, the patient may decide to move bedtime to 11.30 p.m. and/or get-up time to 6.30 a.m. This process is continued until the amount of sleep he requires is reached and regular sleep and get-up time is maintained.

Sometimes restriction of time in bed can be difficult to implement and medication can initially be used to help in the process.

Suggestions for better sleep

1 Go to bed only when you are sleepy.

2 Don't use your bed for anything except sleep and sexual activity.

3 If you are unable to fall asleep, get up and go into another room. Stay up as long as you wish, preferably engaged in a boring activity. Go back to bed only when you feel sleepy. Although you should not watch the clock, the goal is to fall asleep quickly; if you are in bed for more than ten minutes without falling asleep, you should get out of bed.

4 Repeat step 3 as often as necessary throughout the night.

5 Set your alarm and get up at the same time each day, regardless of how much sleep you got during the night.

6 Don't take naps during the day; it will interfere with your ability to fall asleep at night.

7 Avoid caffeinated beverages (coffee, tea and colas) in the evening.

8 Avoid excessive liquids in the evening, in order to minimise the need for nighttime trips to the bathroom.

9 The chronic use of tobacco disturbs sleep.

10 Avoid heavy physical exercise in the evening.

11 Avoid alcohol, especially in the evening. Although alcohol helps people to fall asleep, the resulting sleep is fragmented.

12 People who feel angry and frustrated because they cannot sleep should not try harder and harder to fall asleep, but should get out of bed, go to another room and do something different.

13 If you find that you look at the clock at night, turn it so you cannot see it or cover it up.

Sleep should not be judged on a day-by-day basis

It should be strongly emphasised that sleep quality varies over time, like any other body function. Waking up each morning and asking yourself if you had a good night's sleep should be avoided. It is a useless exercise that tends to increase the level of anxiety.

Sleep quality should be assessed together with daytime function over an extended period, perhaps four or five weeks.

Understanding the underlying mechanism of psychophysiological insomnia

It is important to become aware of the events and emotions that trigger and maintain insomnia. This can be a difficult process and may need expert help. As a protective mechanism, people can sometimes minimise or completely deny events and emotions; however, these should be fully evaluated if insomnia is to be dealt with.

Medications

Medications are useful when used at the right time and in the right context. In transient insomnia during stressful periods, sleeping tablets with short or medium action—six to eight hours (Temazepam, Imovan™)—can be useful to help the person through. On rare occasions in chronic insomnia, medications need to be continued for a long time. This may be the case when other strategies fail or are not feasible. However, there is no demonstrated evidence to support benefit from continued use of sleeping tablets apart from subjective reports. In this situation the use of medication *'when needed'*, perhaps once or twice a week, is an acceptable compromise.

This is a similar strategy used in other chronic conditions. For example, people with severe daily migraine need daily medication. Similarly, patients with severe pain due to osteoporosis may need morphine daily to manage their symptoms.

✷ Getting old and insomnia

A complaint of insomnia is more common in old age and there are many reasons for it.

Sleep changes with age

Figure 3 (see Chapter 1) shows how quantity and structure of sleep changes as we get older. With age, sleep is more superficial, with increased arousals, less deep sleep (slow wave sleep) and less REM sleep. The distinction between sleep and wake becomes more blurred, with naps taken through the day. Some sleep disorders such as restless legs, periodic limb movement disorder and sleep apnoea are common in the elderly and contribute to sleep fragmentation and insomnia.

Social changes

Retirement brings about changes in daily life. Routines such as bedtime, get-up time, commuting to work, and mealtimes, which have been stable for many years, are no longer dictated by work commitments. The level of physical and mental activity may be substantially reduced. The person has to go through a process of readjustment of their role in society and within the family.

Medical and psychiatric illnesses

Elderly people are more likely to have medical problems and to be on multiple medications.

Depression is also common in the elderly. This is sometimes the result of chronic medical illnesses which reduce the person's function, the loss of family members and their change of role in society. Elderly people living in hostels or nursing homes are particularly at risk of insomnia, because many of the factors mentioned above are likely to be present. They are often on multiple medications; they have poor mobility; and they are indoors for prolonged periods with scanty exposure to sunlight. They are often subject to rigid timetables, with meals served early and early bedtime. In some elderly people, disturbed sleep is symptomatic of worsening mental function (dementia). The use of sleeping tablets and antidepressants is common in nursing homes, causing daytime drowsiness and further reduction in physical and mental activity.

Treatment

Treatment needs to take all of the above factors into account. Optimisation of medical treatment, psychological counselling, and promotion of regular physical and mental activity are paramount. Review of medications and their interactions, and limiting prescriptions to only essential drugs, is also very important.

'Sleeping tablets are bad for you and you should not use them.' This is a common theme discussed in the media, and one espoused by many medical professionals.

It is clearly stated in this chapter that sleeping tablets are not an answer to insomnia. Sleeping tablets cannot overcome the sadness, the pain and the sense of guilt following the death of a son. Sleeping tablets cannot overcome the sense of solitude and isolation that some elderly people experience. However, we also see people who are in their seventies or eighties referred to our unit who have been on sleeping tablets of one kind or another for many years, sometimes for half their life! In some of these people, taking these tablets at night was perhaps the only way they were able to cope with different situations in life. Even worse, prescription of the tablets was the only advice they received from the medical professional who lacked the time or the skill to provide counselling.

Table 5.1   Medications and Insomnia

Medication	Comment
Theophylline	Used in asthma (Theo-Dur™, Neulin™, Austyn™)
Nasal decongestant	Often they contain vasoconstrictors that are a stimulant—such as ephedrine, pseudo-ephedrine (Sudafed™, Sinutab™, Tylenol cold & Flu™, etc.)
Coffee	More than 3–4 cups per day are likely to interfere with sleep, but the effect varies from one person to another
Alcohol	Causes awakening and fragmentation of sleep in the second part of the night
Nicotine	Is a stimulant
'Old' antidepressants (Tricyclic)	Can exacerbate periodic limb movements during sleep and cause daytime sleepiness (Deptran™, Endep™, Anafranil™, Prothiaden™)
'New' antidepressants (MAOIs, SSRIs)	Can cause insomnia (Aurorix™, Prozac™, Aropax™, Zoloft™)
Sleeping tablets	Can cause muscle relaxation and insomnia by worsening sleep apnoea
Blood pressure tablets	Can cause insomnia by acting on the nervous system (Catapress™, Tenormin™, Betaloc™, Inderal™, Aldomet™)
Fluid tablets	Can cause insomnia because of the urge to pass water in the middle of the night (Lasix™, Urex™, Moduretic™, Dapa-Tabs™, Diulo™)
Antibiotic	Quinolone (Ciproxin™, Noroxin™) are suggested to cause insomnia
Anti-cholesterol agents (anti-lipid)	The 'Vastin' (Lipex™, Zocor™) group are reported to cause drowsiness and fatigue
Anti-Parkinson medication	L-dopa, bromocriptine, amantadine can cause insomnia
Thyroid hormones	Oroxine if in excess can cause insomnia
Cortisone	Decadron™, Sone™, Panafcort™ etc. can cause insomnia in some patients

These patients are often well adjusted and don't feel they have a problem, except when they are told that taking sleeping tablets is bad for them and they start to feel guilty about taking them. Our advice in this situation is practical: sleeping tablets are like any other medication: not bad, not good. Use them when needed.

Table 5.1 shows how medications used for other medical conditions can affect sleep in different ways.

6

Sleepiness, tiredness and fatigue

- People often use *fatigue* and *tiredness* as a proxy for *sleepiness*.
- Fatigue, tiredness and sleepiness are non-specific symptoms.
- Sleep deprivation is one of the most common causes of chronic tiredness in an otherwise healthy person.
- Our body never adjusts to shift work.
- Investigation of chronic fatigue needs consideration of three main areas (metabolic/inflammatory, psychiatric, and sleep–wake function disorders).
- Narcoleptic syndromes are often not diagnosed for years, with significant suffering for the patient. Treatment is available.

Chronic tiredness and fatigue are common symptoms and are reported by up to one in four patients presenting to a general practitioner. *Tiredness* refers to a lack of energy. *Fatigue* and *fatigability* are defined as tiring abnormally early during prolonged activity, be it physical, mental or both. *Sleepiness* refers to the desire to lie down and go to sleep.

Because of the widely held view of the restorative function of sleep, sleepiness is often regarded as a consequence of being tired. Often people say, 'I'm so tired that I need to go to sleep', meaning that they fall asleep because they need to recover their energy. People often use the terms *tiredness* and *fatigue* to mean physical and mental fatigue, but also sleepiness. This way of thinking is not necessarily true. A person can be physically exhausted but be unable to go to sleep. Or they can be sleepy without having engaged in any exhausting physical or mental activity. Of course, a person can be tired, fatigued and sleepy at the same time.

These distinctions between tiredness, fatigue and sleepiness are important in understanding the underlying mechanism in people in whom fatigue becomes a major symptom—in particular, in people with chronic fatigue syndrome.

❋ Understanding and investigating people with chronic fatigue and sleepiness

Fatigue is a common symptom of many illnesses but specific of none. This is to say that there may be many possible causes of persistent fatigue.

Figure 19 shows the three main areas that need to be considered.

Metabolic/endocrine/inflammatory/autoimmune conditions

There are many common—and less common—conditions in which chronic fatigue can be the presenting symptom. Metabolic and endocrine disorders such as iron deficiency, vitamin B12 and folate deficiency, thyroid hormone dysfunction, anaemia and diabetes are common examples.

Chronic inflammation due to bacteria or viruses, or resulting from an abnormal immune response such as hepatitis,

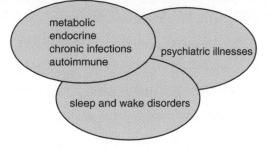

Figure 19 Causes of chronic fatigue

rheumatoid arthritis, lupus and related conditions, needs to be considered. Many medications used today can also be responsible for chronic fatigue and tiredness, as well as sleepiness.

Psychiatric illnesses

Patients with depression and anxiety disorders can complain of fatigue and tiredness. Fatigue in psychiatric illnesses often has a connotation of lack of drive and motivation. The severity of patients' symptoms can fluctuate with time. Sleep–wake cycle disorders are common in psychiatric illness and are part of the illness itself.

The majority of medications used by psychiatrists can also cause the same symptoms as side-effects. This applies to the antidepressants as well as to the benzodiazepines commonly used in these conditions.

Sleep–wake cycle disorders

This is a major group which is often neglected in the investigation of fatigue and tiredness unless the patient specifically complains of sleepiness. However, often the patient uses the term *tiredness* not only to describe physical and mental fatigue but also sleepiness, because sleepiness—the desire to lie down and close one's eyes—is interpreted as a consequence of being tired.

In previous chapters we have seen that common sleep disorders such as sleep apnoea, periodic limb movement disorder and delayed sleep phase syndrome can all cause tiredness and sleepiness during the day. Here we consider some less appreciated and less well-known conditions:

- chronic sleep deprivation and shift working;
- narcolepsy and its variants;
- chronic fatigue syndrome; and
- jet lag.

❋ Chronic sleep deprivation and shift working

Chronic sleep deprivation is perhaps the most common and *underestimated* cause of daytime tiredness and sleepiness. Two important points need to be clarified:

- Sleep loss accumulates over time.
- Healthy people have large physical and mental reserves that allow them to cope for a long time with sleep deprivation.

A sleep loss of thirty minutes or an hour a day can be well tolerated, but it does accumulate over time. A person can easily adjust to small amounts of sleep loss which can last for months or years, because of their large physical and mental reserves that allow them to maintain a good level of performance. However, after a certain period of time, which can vary in different individuals, reserves can run out and symptoms of fatigue, sleepiness and ill-health become apparent.

This set of events makes it difficult for some people to connect sleep deprivation due to shift working or a particular lifestyle with the onset of fatigue and tiredness. The person might have been a shift worker for ten years and able to manage reasonably well before symptoms become important and affect his or her well-being to the point of seeking medical advice.

Irregular work hours and shift working are always associated with some degree of tiredness and sleepiness. This applies to all forms of shifting, be it eight-hour or twelve-hour shifts, or early morning shifts (starting work between 4 and 7 a.m.). Approximately two out of ten night workers report falling asleep regularly at work. A recent survey of long haul truck drivers in the United States showed periods of drowsiness while driving, particularly at night, even though these episodes did not result in motor vehicle accidents.

It is interesting to note that even people who are 'on call' suffer from disrupted sleep.

Sleep deprivation, with the consequent daytime drowsiness, fatigue and reduction in attention span, is likely to be one of the causes of job-related accidents. This is particularly important at nighttime. Major disasters such as the Three Mile Island and Chernobyl nuclear power incidents, and the oil spill of the tanker *Exxon Valdez*, all occurred at night and human fatigue may have been a contributing factor.

There is a lot of uncertainty regarding the implications of shift working because studies are difficult to perform. However, some general comments can be made and some misconceptions clarified.

During shift work, and in particular night work, sleepiness occurs because of *overall loss of sleep* and because *body rhythms* are out of phase. The view that permanent night shift and slow shift rotation (seven days on day shift, seven on afternoon shift and seven on night shift) minimise or overcome this problem is incorrect, because the biological rhythm of permanent night workers never adjusts completely to night shift. Short rotating shifts (two to three days) may result in an improved sense of well-being compared to slow rotating or permanent night shift. The direction of shift rotation may also be important. Because the body rhythm tends to be slightly longer than 24 hours, close to 25 hours on average, the body tends to slightly prolong the day, and forward rotation (day, afternoon, night) may be better tolerated.

In the search for increased productivity and efficiency, twelve-hour shifts have become more common. Available evidence indicates that performance deteriorates as fatigue increases. The degree of sleep deprivation and consequent fatigue becomes particularly severe when workers are requested to do an extra half a shift or a double shift. This is common in situations where there is a need to increase productivity to meet deadlines, and where the tendency is to increase working hours instead of recruiting more workers.

In modern society, sleep deprivation is also present in non-shift workers. Overtime, with its economic reward, is common in all jobs. If commuting time is taken into consideration, the working day of many people is a standard ten hours. Some people may have a second job or study part-time. On top of all this, there are family, social and recreational activities for which time must be found, and usually sleep and resting time is sacrificed with resulting sleep deprivation.

Although sleep requirements vary from one person to another, it is well established that less than five hours' sleep on average is associated with sleep deprivation in the majority of people. This results in an increase in levels of sleepiness and tiredness. In this respect, teenagers have been shown to be particularly at risk because of irregular sleep and wake habits.

Management of sleep deprivation

The first step is recognising that chronic sleep deprivation is the cause of tiredness/sleepiness and related complications such as poor memory or concentration, mood changes and, sometimes, personal crises. A connection between lifestyle and tiredness is often not made and on occasion is resisted. Adoption of regular sleep habits to increase rest time is recommended. For some people this may mean giving up some activities that are not essential. The following is a good example.

A thirty-year-old woman was seen because of chronic fatigue and sleepiness of twelve months' duration. She decided to seek help for her problem because recently she had started to nod off while driving to work. She is a veterinary nurse who works eight hours a day, six days a week, with two hours a day commuting time. She attends university for two hours, two nights a week and studies for a further eight hours a week.

She also runs a dog training session one evening a week and attends to her weekly house chores, including her own pets. In her 'spare time' she edits and publishes a newsletter for children on how to care for pets.

The patient was deprived of sleep because of the number of activities she had taken on. She needed to reduce these in order to allow more time for resting and sleeping. She also considered the possibility of finding a job closer to home, as this would save her two hours of commuting each day.

Much more difficult is to find solutions when the sleep deprivation is 'built in' in work practices like shift working. Some suggestions can be made on an individual level to minimise the negative effect. However, the problem requires social awareness, and political and industrial relations decisions on work practices, safety in the workplace and protection of workers' well-being.

A standard work shift plus overtime should be avoided. In occupations at high risk, such as truck drivers, the number of hours a person can drive needs to be regulated by law because the bargaining power of individual drivers, who may face the prospect of losing their job, is very limited.

Current knowledge suggests that the time of day when sleep is taken is important. Nighttime sleep is needed for a person to be refreshed. The best sleep appears to be obtained when started between 9 p.m. and 1 a.m.

It takes at least two consecutive nights' sleep to recover from a night shift. Therefore, two or three days of night shift should be followed by at least two days off. The belief that the body adjusts to *continuous* night work is not true.

Napping on the job

Napping has been proposed as a strategy to improve alertness and performance during prolonged activity and night work. Napping for twenty minutes to a few hours improves alertness and performance. This is already implemented in the transportation industry where truck drivers are required to have a 'rest period' every few hours when driving and to keep a record of these breaks in their log book. The beneficial effect of napping has also been shown in the performance of pilots in transpacific flights under experimental conditions.

Use of bright light and medications

The light and darkness cycle is the most powerful factor influencing sleep and wakefulness. Exposure to a well-lit environment during night work and shielding from light during daytime sleep is a useful measure which can help workers to cope with a rotating shift. The use of short-acting sleeping tablets such as triazolam, zopiclone, zolpidem and temazepam can also help the worker to adjust to a new roster in the first or second sleep period after the beginning of a night shift. The use of melatonin, with its sleep-promoting effect, has also been investigated in this setting.

✳ Excessive daytime sleepiness (narcolepsy and its variants)

The term *narcolepsy* is derived from Greek and literally means *falling asleep*. There are many other terms used to describe conditions of excess sleepiness, such as *abnormal REM sleep*, *non-REM narcolepsy* and *hypersomnia*. If sleepiness started after a severe head trauma, usually associated with unconsciousness, it is sometimes called *post-traumatic hypersomnia*. Brain tumours can also present as narcoleptic syndrome (secondary narcolepsy).

For simplicity we will refer to this group of conditions as narcoleptic syndromes. There are different symptoms that may be present in narcoleptic syndromes, but one that is *always* present is sleepiness/tiredness.

Sleepiness and tiredness in narcoleptic syndromes

Patients with narcolepsy can have different degrees of daytime sleepiness and tiredness. Some have a history of an irresistible need to fall asleep. The patient falls asleep for ten or twenty minutes and then is able to resume his or her activities to full capacity. This may be repeated many times through the day.

In other people, however, the feeling is more one of a sub-wakefulness state during which the patient can fall asleep at any time if given the opportunity. This often happens if the patient is engaged in a boring activity such as driving, reading or watching television, or travelling as a passenger in a car. Some people describe the feeling as a thick fog hanging over their head which they are unable to shake off completely. Some people with narcoleptic syndrome can nap for two or three hours and still wake up unrefreshed.

In some patients, but not all, nighttime sleep is restless and broken, and the person wakes up in the morning feeling unrefreshed.

The symptoms of narcolepsy can start at any age from childhood to old age. However, they usually start around the teenage years and during the forties. Often people with narcoleptic syndrome are not diagnosed for a long time. Some are labelled as 'lazy' or 'a sleepy head'. If the condition started in childhood, they often have problems learning and may drop out of school at an early age. They then have difficulty keeping a job, because they are always late and don't perform well. Patients with narcoleptic syndrome often have a history of car accidents, as well as an increased risk of workplace accidents. Usually there is a long history of symptoms going back many years, on average fifteen years, before the diagnosis is made. Some people manage to put in place coping mechanisms. For example, they try to take a nap whenever an opportunity arises, such as during their lunch break or while sitting as a passenger in a car. People with narcolepsy and increased sleepiness tendency have frequent depressive symptoms, personal and interpersonal problems, and work difficulties. Sleepiness and tiredness in narcoleptic syndrome *need not be continuous*. The severity of symptoms can fluctuate over time.

The following symptoms are also seen in people with narcolepsy.

Cataplexy

Cataplexy refers to a sudden loss of power in any muscle group in the body which can occur particularly during strong emotions such as when laughing, or feeling frustrated, surprised, angry or scared. At times it is described as a 'jelly-like feeling' going through the body which can last from half a second to a few minutes. It becomes particularly obvious if it involves leg muscles, in which case the person has the feeling of buckling at the knees or ankles and could even fall to the ground—not because the person loses consciousness, but because their muscles don't hold them up. Cataplexy is due to the intrusion of REM-brain activity during wakefulness. As the body muscles lose their tone (strength) during REM, the person experiences muscle weakness while awake.

Strictly speaking, the word *narcolepsy* should be reserved for people with a combination of irresistible sleep attacks and the presence of cataplexy. However, the presence of cataplexy is rare. There is a larger group of people who have an increased sleepiness tendency/tiredness that is not totally disabling and who do not have cataplexy.

Sleep paralysis

Sleep paralysis is seen frequently in narcoleptic syndrome, but also in other conditions where sleepiness/tiredness is present. People with sleep apnoea and periodic limb movement disorder can also report sleep paralysis. Sleep paralysis occurs when the person is going to sleep or waking up from sleep. The person is awake but has the feeling of being unable to move. This sensation tends to end on its own after a few seconds or can be terminated by a touch from another person or a sound from the environment. Sleep paralysis is associated with unpleasant feelings and is often frightening. It occurs when the person wakes up from REM sleep and is due to a delay in regaining muscle strength when the brain has already woken up.

Hypnagogic and hypnopompic hallucinations

These hallucinations are also common in narcolepsy but, like sleep paralysis, are not exclusive to it. *Hypnagogic* (at the beginning of sleep) and *hypnopompic* (at the end of sleep) *hallucinations* refer to a dream state occurring when the person is half awake during which they have vivid, brightly coloured hallucinations. The abnormal feeling can be visual or auditory (hearing voices or noises), or even a feeling of abnormal body position or an 'extra corporeal' experience.

Although the symptoms of sleepiness and tiredness are always present in narcolepsy, the other symptoms may or may not be present, or may be present for a brief period of time but not later on in life. Some people report having experienced hypnagogic hallucinations or sleep paralysis only once or twice in their life-time.

Mechanisms of excessive sleepiness/tiredness in narcoleptic syndromes

In sleep disorders such as sleep apnoea and periodic limb movement disorder, sleepiness during the day is the result of poor sleep quality and fragmentation at night. In narcoleptic syndrome the problem is due to abnormal regulation of the sleep–wake function, which is a 24-hour function and modulated by light and night cycling. The sleepiness tendency that is normal at night tends to spill over into the daytime and wakefulness tends to intrude at nighttime. As mentioned above, the symptoms can be dramatic, to the point where the person has the irresistible need to fall asleep for a few minutes, or they can be more subtle and less severe.

Treatment of narcoleptic syndromes

The most important step is to recognise that the tiredness in people with sleep–wake cycle disorders is closely linked to an increase in sleepiness tendency. This link is often missed for many years, and the average time between the onset of symptoms and diagnosis is about fifteen years.

Once the diagnosis is made, the person may need no treatment at all if the symptoms are mild and they do not work in a high-risk occupation. Regular naps through the day are a possible option, which reduces sleepiness through the day. If this is not possible because of lifestyle or if it is not sufficient, treatment with stimulant medication during the day usually provides some symptomatic relief. In narcoleptic syndrome the balance between wakefulness and sleepiness is in favour of sleepiness and the stimulant medications are used to increase the level of alertness. This results in better functioning during the day, both physically and mentally, as well as improving sleep quality at night.

Current medications available in Australia include dexamphetamine and Ritalin® These are amphetamine-like medications and require special approval for their prescription. Stimulant medications do not cure narcoleptic syndrome but only provide symptomatic relief. There are many issues associated with their use and these are discussed in Chapter 8. It should be stressed that, even when treated, people with narcolepsy remain more sleepy than normal subjects.

Modafinil is a non-amphetamine stimulant shown to be as effective as dexamphetamine in narcolepsy. It is available in Europe and the United States but not yet in Australia (see Chapter 8). Other medications used in narcolepsy include gamma-hydroxybutyrate, ritanserin, pemoline and viloxazine. However, they are not as effective as dexamphetamine, Ritalin™ and modafinil.

✳ Chronic fatigue syndrome

Patients with chronic fatigue syndrome (CFS) constitute a diverse group of people in whom the main symptom is *self-reported fatigue of at least six months' duration for which no other causes have been found*. As this definition implies, CFS is unlikely to be a disease on its own. It is more often the end-result of different conditions, some of which have been discovered and have been excluded from the definition, and others that are unknown but are lumped together under the name of chronic fatigue syndrome. One difficulty in patients with CFS is that no obvious abnormalities are found by conventional medical examination.

People with symptoms of chronic fatigue have been recognised for more than a hundred years and different names have been used for the condition. Towards the end of the nineteenth century the word *neuro-asthenia* was used. Neuro-asthenia literally means 'weakness of the nervous system'.

It was felt that although nothing abnormal could be found, the symptoms may have been due to some abnormality of the nervous system.

At the beginning of the twentieth century the term *psycho-asthenia* (weakness of the psyche) was used by some, suggesting that symptoms of chronic fatigue may have been due to some emotional lability.

At times, chronic fatigue has appeared in clusters of individuals working in the same environment. In England, the term *myalgic encephalomyelitis* (ME) has been used, even though no evidence of encephalitis (inflammation of the brain) has ever been found. The term is no longer used.

In the 1980s the possibility of CFS being related to immune system dysfunction led to use of the term *chronic fatigue and immune dysfunction syndrome*. It is now clear that, although the immune system may play a role in the origin of the symptoms, it is not responsible for chronic fatigue in its own right.

An international meeting held in Dublin in 1994 concluded that the term *chronic fatigue syndrome* should be used and that an effort should be made to identify subgroups of patients who may share similar features within the larger group of CFS patients. In patients with CFS and who have marked muscle aches, the term *fibromyalgia* is often used.

Symptoms of chronic fatigue syndrome

In about one-third of patients, fatigue started suddenly following what appeared to be a 'flu-like' illness. Some infections are well known, such as glandular fever, Ross River virus, Q fever, cytomegalovirus infection and Lyme disease, but in many patients a specific diagnosis is not made. Exposure to some toxins seems to be the starting event in some. Ciguatera poisoning is a documented association.

Ciguatera is caused by eating certain fish from temperate waters. The toxin, ciguatoxin, is resistant to boiling, salting, freezing or cooking so ciguatera poisoning can be contracted far away from tropical and sub-tropical areas where the fish were caught. Ciguatoxin has no unusual smell or taste and is not related to how fresh the fish is. The toxin is produced by microscopic organisms associated with algae. It is passed from small fish that eat algae to larger carnivorous fish and from these to humans. Ciguatera poisoning can be contracted through many types of fish. In Australia it has been reported in mackerel, coral trout, grouper, red schnapper, yellow tail and kingfish among others. During acute ciguatera poisoning the person can experience pins and needles around the mouth, feelings of hot and cold, diarrhoea, vomiting, aches and pains in the muscles and joints, skin rash and itch. Symptoms usually resolve without any specific treatment. However, in some patients even after weeks or months, fatigue, tiredness, lethargy and muscle pain persist.

Exposure to other toxins such as organochlorines and organophosphates has been reported as a possible cause of chronic fatigue, but there is no scientific evidence for it.

Patients with chronic fatigue often have memory and concentration problems, muscle and joint aches and pains, new onset of headaches and post-exertion malaise. Symptoms of depression and anxiety are also common.

The majority of patients which CFS report sleep disturbances, from difficulty initiating and maintaining sleep to feeling unrefreshed despite prolonged hours of sleep.

Sleep–wake cycle in chronic fatigue syndrome

As mentioned in Chapter 1, sleep and wake function is part of the autonomic nervous system. This is the system that regulates functions in our body that are not under our direct control. Examples are digestion, kidney function, blood pressure control, sweating, hormonal function (for example, menstrual regulation) and breathing. If we eat something, digestion will start irrespective of whether we want it to or not. Even if we don't think about breathing, we still breathe. Sleep and wake tendency is also part of the autonomic nervous system and is strongly regulated by light and night cycling. In at least a subgroup of patients with CFS, a disturbance of the sleep and wake system is likely to be responsible for chronic fatigue, both in terms of lack of energy, physical and mental exhaustion and increased sleepiness tendency.

People with CFS have many other symptoms that point towards dysfunction of the autonomic nervous system. Apart from tiredness, they often report low or unstable blood pressure, irritable bowel symptoms, menstrual irregularity and inappropriate sweating. The areas of the brain that regulate sleep and wake also regulate the other functions of the autonomic nervous system. The brain stem, hypothalamus and limbic system (Figure 20) are the parts of the brain involved in these activities. Interestingly, the same area and nearby

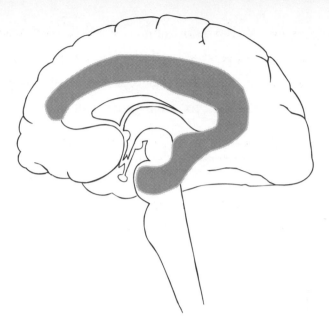

Figure 20   The limbic system (shaded area)

structures are also important for functions such as memory, which is often impaired in chronic fatigue.

The observation that at least some patients with CFS have a disturbance of wake and sleep function is important because of treatment implications. When patients with chronic fatigue are asked the question, 'What do you mean by fatigue? Do you mean lack of energy, that everything you do is an extra effort? Do you mean the desire to put your head down and have a sleep? or do you mean lack of drive, lack of motivation, a "couldn't be bothered" kind of feeling?', the majority respond that it is a combination of all three but the lack of energy is the most important symptom. Yet when they are studied with an overnight polysomnography and day-time naps (multiple sleep latency test), they often show increased daytime sleepiness tendency with abnormalities of

REM similar to narcolepsy patients. This indicates that at least some symptoms may be due to a decreased level of alertness, the balance of sleep and wake being in favour of sleepiness. The patients often refer to this sensation as *tiredness and fatigue*.

Based on this interpretation, some of our patients with CFS are treated with small doses of stimulant medication during the day similar to narcoleptic patients, to increase their level of alertness. The results of empirical application of this treatment are encouraging, and proper studies are under way to confirm this hypothesis.

✳ Jet lag

The availability of fast transport such as aircraft, and their use by millions of people, has made jet lag a common problem. This is particularly the case for transoceanic flights, when the time difference can be eight to ten hours. In this situation our biological clock is still tuned to the home time, but the body has to adjust to and function according to the new local time. For instance, when flying from Sydney to Rome, there is a time difference of ten hours. When it is 3 p.m. in Rome, our internal clock feels like it is 1 a.m. at home. When it is 11 p.m. in Rome and we are supposed to be ready to go to sleep, our internal clock is at 9 a.m., ready to wake up and start the day. The result is a variety of symptoms that include difficulty initiating and maintaining sleep, decreased performance, lack of concentration, general malaise, dull headache, abdominal discomfort and lack of appetite.

The body eventually adjusts to the new environment, but it takes approximately one day for each hour difference. It is recognised that adaptation is faster when flying westward than eastward. This is due to the fact that our internal clock tends to be closer to 25 hours than 24 hours and therefore the tendency is to prolong the day, as is the case when we are flying westward. The reverse is true flying eastward. It is also true that individuals vary in their ability to adjust to a new time zone.

Management of jet lag

The body will adjust to time zone change, but we can help to speed up the process. The airlines tend to schedule their meals and entertainment activity in tune with the time at the port of destination. Meals are important environmental cues that help to time our body functions. However, the more important cue is light and dark cycling. So, when you arrive at a new destination, exposure to natural light during the day is very important to speed up the adjustment of the internal clock. The avoidance of naps during the day is also important.

Going back to our example of a trip from Sydney to Rome, if the arrival is scheduled for morning, the usual time, it could be useful to use short-acting sleeping tablets soon after leaving Bangkok or Singapore to try and get at least a few hours of sleep. Melatonin also appears to be promising in helping to reset the clock to the new location. The use of 0.3–1 milligram of melatonin for three days in the evening helps to speed up the body's adjustment to a new time zone.

�֍ Endozepine stupor

This is the name given to a condition of prolonged drowsiness, which has defied understanding until recently. The following example is typical of this condition.

A 51-year-old man was referred for assessment of recurrent episodes which started with the patient feeling irritable and very fatigued. He would put himself to bed or fall asleep on the lounge. His wife could not wake him up. With strong stimulation he might become less drowsy and would be able to go to the toilet, but he would refuse any food. If the stimulation persisted, he might become abusive and aggressive. The episodes initially lasted for two to three days, but more recently for only one day. The patient eventually became more responsive and gradually regained full awareness of his surroundings. He had no recollection of the events. The attacks occurred with a variable frequency of between twice a month and three times a year. All the investigations were normal, including physical examination, CT (computed tomography) and MRI (magnetic resonance imaging) of the head, EEG and blood tests.

Patients with a similar presentation have recently been studied in depth in Europe and were found to have a high level of endozepine–4. Endozepines are substances produced by the body that act like benzodiazepines (the diazepam group). They are similar to the more widely known endorphins. Endorphins are the body's equivalent of morphine, and the endozepines are the body's equivalent of the benzodiazepines. It is hypothesised that a high level of these substances causes the patient to become deeply asleep, almost in a light coma. It is not known why this happens. However, the use of flumazenil, a medication that blocks the action of the endozepine, wakes the patients immediately. Unfortunately, the effect of flumazenil lasts only ten to fifteen minutes and needs to be given intravenously. Attempts to use a formulation by mouth to prevent the attacks have had little success. This condition is probably more frequent than is currently recognised. The attacks may be labelled *psychogenic* or *hysterical* (as in the patient in the example). Awareness of these symptoms may point the patient and the family in the right direction.

7

Children and sleep

- Children are not small adults.
- In the first twelve months of life, children need to 'learn' to sleep.
- Allowing for differences between children, most bedtime problems stem from lack of consistency in the parents' behaviour.
- Parents need to set and implement bedtime 'limits' with reassuring firmness.
- Sleep apnoea in children is different from apnoea in adults. Daytime sleepiness is not common in childhood sleep apnoea.
- Adolescents have an increased sleep tendency, but often get less sleep than required.

When medical students start their training in paediatric medicine the first thing they are told is that 'children are not small adults'. This neatly summarises the important point that the anatomy, function and disorders in children are different from those in adults, and this is particularly true for sleep and wake function.

Some sleep disturbances such as snoring, sleep apnoea, sleep walking and narcolepsy are shared by children and adults, but the presenting symptoms are often different in the two groups.

With infants and toddlers, behavioural problems are a

common symptom of sleep disorders. They are the source of distress and emotional conflict within the family, as well as causing sleep disruption for the parents.

Adolescence is a period of great social, personal and hormonal changes, and sleep is no exception.

We will review here aspects of sleep disorders that are more typical of children. Other conditions that are also common in childhood, such as sleep walking and sleep terrors are discussed in Chapter 4.

✳ Learning to sleep

Sleep in infants (less than twelve months of age) differs markedly from sleep in adults, both in terms of organisation and structure in relation to sleep stages. At about 32 weeks of gestation it is possible to identify two states of sleep, called *active sleep* and *quiet sleep*, that are considered equivalent to REM sleep and non-REM sleep respectively. During active sleep there are frequent eye movements, and movements involving the face and body. During quiet sleep, respiration becomes regular and motor activity ceases. The distinction between active and quiet sleep is often blurred, and a third stage, called *intermediate sleep*, is often seen.

Infants can go directly from wakefulness into REM sleep, unlike adults, whose sleep onset occurs through non-REM sleep. At four to six months of age, non-REM sleep starts becoming more structured and the Stages 1, 2, 3 and 4 can now be recognised, similar to the adult pattern, in keeping with maturation of the brain.

Newborns spend an average of sixteen hours a day sleeping, alternating three to four hours' sleep with one to two hours of wakefulness usually coupled with feeding across the 24 hours. By three months, sleep is reduced to fourteen hours a day, and a day/night pattern starts emerging with a lengthening of the sleep episode at night. At the end of the first year, a nighttime pattern of sleep is established and daytime sleep assumes the features of napping.

The number of naps and the time spent napping also decrease with age. It is normal for toddlers and pre-school children to nap once a day unless family or their social schedule prevents it. It should be stressed that napping at four to five years of age is not only normal but should not be discouraged. In this age group, sleep obtained during afternoon naps appears to be structurally different from night sleep, with an increase in deep sleep (Stage 4) which may be functionally important in the 24-hour balance of sleep and complements nighttime sleep.

By the time children start school, the amount of sleep is further reduced to nine to ten hours. Napping becomes rarer.

At puberty the amount of sleep obtained by adolescents suffers a marked decline, to less than seven or eight hours. It is difficult to be sure how much this reduction is a reflection of hormonal and maturational changes and how much it depends on social factors (such as staying up late at night, going to parties, and the use of recreational drugs, including alcohol).

The development of sleep and wake function from infancy to early adulthood is subject to individual variability. It can be disrupted along the way, with important effects on the physical and emotional well-being of the child and the parents. It can also be argued that it may set a pattern, which becomes long-standing and persists in adulthood.

✳ Difficulty getting to sleep and staying asleep in infants and toddlers

Difficulty with sleep onset and sleep maintenance is the main area of sleep complaints in the parents of infants and toddlers. Parents who have to struggle with their children at bedtime and during the night often exhibit symptoms of anxiety, distress and occasional violence.

There are two groups of causes to consider:

- medical; and
- behavioural (the majority).

For both groups of conditions, close contact with and help from the family doctor or counsellor are needed.

Medical causes

It is important that medical conditions that can cause distress to the child are excluded. Gastro-oesophageal reflux, asthma and ear infections are frequent causes of sleep disruption and need specific treatment. A 'colicky baby' is an otherwise healthy infant who has frequent bouts of inconsolable crying. Although crying is a universal occurrence in the first twelve months of life, a subgroup of babies tend to have frequent bouts of crying. It usually starts in the first two weeks after birth and tends to resolve after three months. The reason is unclear, but it may be related to abnormal response to stimuli such as changes in temperature and digestive difficulties. Although crying can occur anytime during the day, it tends to be more frequent in the evening and reduces in 80 per cent of infants after midnight. It is most distressing for the parents, who try all sorts of remedies to soothe the distressed child. They try different strategies such as feeding and sucking, rhythmic motions such as rocking the baby, cuddles and even car rides around town. These manoeuvres are usually unsuccessful. However, because the bouts of crying often end with the infant asleep, an association with the above soothing activities and falling asleep may develop and persist even after age three to four months when the 'colic' eventually resolves. The use of medications is not recommended. The parents need help in understanding the nature of the problem to make sure that the colicky baby of the first three months does not become a baby with difficulties falling asleep and staying asleep in the following months.

It should be emphasised that 'colic' occurs in healthy babies with no other symptoms. The occurrence of crying associated either with vomiting, diarrhoea, fast breathing or jerking movements is not due to colic and requires medical assessment.

In the colicky baby the possibility of *cow's milk allergy* needs to be considered, because it presents with similar symptoms and in the first few weeks of life. Cow's milk allergy rapidly improves with the use of a special milk formulation.

Behavioural problems

The first twelve months of life are critical in shaping good sleep and wake habits. Although there appear to be no differences between premature and at term babies, infants who had stressful births, or were born during prolonged and difficult labour, seem to have more disturbed sleep in the following few weeks.

As infants get older they become progressively more aware of their surroundings and reactive to the presence or absence of family faces, such as the mother and father. The mother becomes a reassuring figure, and a stranger can cause fear. Falling asleep may cause separation anxiety. The same applies if the child wakes up and the mother is not there. This is a critical period when infants and young children interact with their parents and develop 'settling' mechanisms and sleep-initiating behaviour which can lead to good sleep habits or be followed by behavioural problems. The above point cannot be over-emphasised, because it is easier to prevent abnormal sleep patterns than to correct them once they are established.

It is important that infants learn to put themselves to sleep. Falling asleep is a learned behaviour and the period between six and twelve months appears to be critical. Babies should be put into their crib or bed *before* falling asleep. If they fall asleep while being nursed, or rocked or fed with a bottle, they then form an association between this pattern and falling asleep. When they wake in the middle of the night, they are unable to return to sleep again unless the 'settling' mechanism is repeated. They signal their needs by crying until the parents come to oblige. Then they fall asleep soon after, while the parents may have difficulty returning to sleep. Even if this happens only a couple of times per night, it is the parents who finish up with a sleep problem.

It is interesting to note that waking up through the night is common in *all children*. Those parents who proudly claim that their children sleep through the night are simply unaware of their children waking, because their children put themselves back to sleep without requesting any intervention.

Although prevention is the preferred option, it is possible to correct sleep onset problems. There are entire books describing strategies ranging from systematic ignoring tactics, a more-or-less gradual withdrawal of parental presence, to the use of medications. Treatment is aimed at teaching infants to relearn how to fall asleep on their own and to find mechanisms of *self-settling*. Making changes gradually is probably the more logical approach. For example, if the child falls asleep only in the presence of the parents, too rapid withdrawal of this association may cause fright and intense separation anxiety, making things more difficult. In such a case the infant should be put in his or her crib when awake and left alone for progressively longer periods, maintaining a reassuring presence in between.

Nocturnal feeding is another association that can perpetuate sleep disruption. Generally, after six months most of the feeding requirements should be obtained through the day. However, in some infants feeding at night continues. The baby may feed a small amount a few times a night, in which case sucking is the main reason for feeding and is a soothing mechanism, as explained above. Other infants feed large quantities with consequent wetting. In this situation, hunger may wake the child through the night. It is as if the pattern of the feeding that is typical of the first few months of life persists, and the establishment of a consolidated sleep at night is delayed.

Treatment consists of slowly decreasing the frequency of feeding, prolonging the intervals between feeds, and reducing the strength of the feed (from full-strength milk to half the strength, and so on) if the child is bottle-fed. If the child is breast-fed, then a progressive reduction in the time of feeding should be implemented.

✳ The question of co-sleeping

This is a controversial issue where parents can get conflicting advice. In Western societies it is often recommended that children should sleep alone in a separate room from a very early age. In other societies and other ethnic groups, having the child in the same room or bed is a normal occurrence. Some studies suggest that children who share their parents' bed regularly have more sleep problems. It is not clear, however, if it is co-sleeping that causes sleep fragmentation, or if children co-sleep because they have a sleep problem. Other studies do not show that co-sleeping is detrimental.

It seems important that the family maintains a consistent behaviour. Allowing the child in the parents' bedroom at times and denying them at other times sends confusing messages to the child. When children have learned to fall asleep on their own at an early age and feel physically and emotionally safe, they can sleep on their own without difficulty.

✳ Head banging and body rocking

Head banging and body rocking are curious behaviours almost exclusive to toddlerhood. The child repeatedly hits the pillow or the bed with his or her head, or moves his or her body from side to side when he or she is drowsy or in a light sleep. The reason for such behaviour is unclear. It is said to be a form of self-gratification used by some children to put themselves to sleep. It is a benign condition that has *no relation* to epilepsy. Padding the side of the bed is sometimes the only measure that is needed.

✳ Bedtime struggles

Bedtime problems become an issue with toddlers and young children. As toddlers pass from the crib to their own bed, they start testing the new situation, sometimes refusing to go to bed in order to maintain contact with their parents. If they go to bed they may delay falling asleep, calling out for more stories, a glass of water, one more kiss good night, or saying they are scared, that they hear something, or that they want to talk about something. The other common behaviour is for the child to settle down in bed for a few minutes and then appear in the lounge-room or parents' bedroom with some request. This behaviour is sometimes referred to as 'curtain calls'. It can be difficult to correct and can test the parents' patience.

There are two main reasons for bedtime difficulties in toddlers and young children:

- limit setting; and
- night fears and anxiety.

Good bedtime habits should be established early on. Children need ten hours of sleep, and a regular pattern needs to be implemented with firmness. Regular activity should be wound down thirty to sixty minutes before bedtime. Teeth brushing, perhaps reading a story or playing with a special object (a favourite blanket, doll or teddy bear) should lead to sleep. Bedtime should be held constant, because if the official bedtime is transgressed with the excuse that homework has to be finished, or the child wants to watch more television or is still hungry, then they will keep testing the limits. This may lead to frustration in the parents. They may start to lose patience and become angry, screaming at the child that they are late for bed. Sometimes the situation is made worse if the child is sharing a room with another sibling. Other times the parents may give in because they think they are responding to real needs (the child is thirsty, hungry or cold). On occasion, marital disagreement or depression may make parenting difficult.

Treatment requires awareness on the parents' part of the need for setting limits and implementing bedtime routine with firmness and consistency. It cannot be over-emphasised that falling asleep is a learned behaviour.

Occasionally, with older toddlers, a reward system may be helpful, such as a star chart or a special object. The variations on this strategy are virtually endless and open to creative solutions, provided the parents are firm in setting and enforcing the child's bedtime.

With young toddlers, particularly at the transition from the crib to the bed, keeping the child in their bedroom may be difficult and the use of a gate at the door to physically prevent the child from coming out may be needed. If this is implemented, reassurance should be given to the child. The parents should stand by the gate without entering the room, so that the child can be reassured of the parents' presence without actually going into the room.

At times, the difficulty in falling asleep is due to fear and stressful events. The child may not be able to express their anxiety directly, but may express their sense of lack of safety by being worried and fearful. Experiences during the day may have been unsettling or interpreted by the child as threatening. There may have been a death in the family, or the child may have started at a new school or the family may have moved to a new home. The child may request to have the lights on or to have parents present in the room. It can be difficult to decide if they are really frightened or if they are using 'fear' to keep the parents in the bedroom.

The issue of whether to keep the bedroom light on is a controversial one. My view is that the light should be turned off as part of sleep onset promoting behaviour, because light is not conducive to sleep. If fear of darkness is intense, a compromise could be to leave a light on in the hallway or a nearby room. The same applies for the presence of the parents. Although this may be allowed initially, it is advisable that the parents gradually withdraw from the room, perhaps to a nearby room so that the child can be reassured of their proximity.

✳ Snoring and disturbed breathing in children

Snoring is common, occurring nightly in one in ten children. The child is usually referred for assessment because the family is concerned by the child's loud snoring or by a noticeable difficulty in breathing. However, a child who snores does not necessarily have sleep apnoea.

As with adults, we can distinguish three conditions:

- primary snoring (snoring only);
- obstructive sleep apnoea; and
- upper airway resistance syndrome.

A child who has *primary snoring* makes the noise, but does not stop breathing (no apnoeas). They are not restless at nighttime and have no daytime symptoms.

The child with *obstructive sleep apnoea* snores most nights (but sleep apnoea may be present with minimal snoring) and has difficulty in breathing, with apnoea lasting from between two and three seconds up to twenty to thirty seconds. The snoring may sometimes have the features of a grunting noise, and the child may appear to be struggling to take in air. The chest may be moving inward and the neck muscles may be tensing up. They tend to be restless through the night, sometimes adopting unusual postures such as extending the neck backwards. Sweating is more common in sleep apnoea. Bed wetting has been quoted to be common, but this is controversial.

In the morning the child is slow to wake up, can be groggy and have a dry mouth. Contrary to adults with sleep apnoea, sleepiness during the day is not common. The child may instead be restless and fidgety, with difficulty maintaining concentration. They can have mood swings, showing unusual aggressiveness as well as social withdrawal and shyness.

When obstructive sleep apnoea is severe, as in the cases of sleep apnoea initially described in the 1970s, it may lead to failure to thrive and heart failure. The presence or absence of the above features helps to distinguish pure snoring from sleep apnoea. However, an overnight sleep study (see Chapter 2) is essential to establish the diagnosis with certainty. When obstructive sleep apnoea is present, the overnight recording shows at least one or more episodes of stopping breathing per hour (in adults, the criteria is five or more episodes per hour), and a drop in oxygen level. In primary snoring these changes do not occur.

Overnight sleep study is also essential to diagnose *upper airway resistance syndrome*. This is similar to the same condition in the adult population (Chapter 3). The child is a snorer and may have all the other features of sleep apnoea, but the overnight recording does not show stopping breathing or oxygen drop.

It is estimated that about two or three out of ten habitual snorers (children who snore every night) have sleep apnoea.

Risk factors for sleep apnoea

Large tonsils and adenoids are the most common risk factor. Obesity increases the risk of sleep apnoea. Between 40 and 50 per cent of children with Down's syndrome are reported to have sleep apnoea which is often not diagnosed. Children with bone and soft tissue of the face abnormalities, such as a small receding chin, a large tongue, cleft palate or achondroplasia, are more likely to have obstructive sleep apnoea.

Sleep apnoea in children is equally common in males and females, contrary to adults where males are four times more likely to suffer from it.

Treatment

No firm statement can be made with regard to treatment. The lack of certainty stems from limited knowledge of the natural progression of snoring and disturbed breathing.

It is uncertain what happens to snoring and sleep apnoea as the child gets older. For instance, snoring is more common with increasing age in adults, but less frequent in children as they grow up. Furthermore, given the fact that large adenoids and tonsils are important factors in sleep apnoea, it is possible that as they become smaller with age, sleep apnoea may resolve spontaneously. So, in mild cases of sleep apnoea (such as minimal daytime symptoms and no significant lack of oxygen), a watch-and-wait approach may be the best option.

The same considerations apply to primary snoring. It is difficult to justify adeno-tonsillectomy (removal of the tonsils and adenoids) and exposing the child to the operative risk because of snoring only. It should also be noted that even a child who is only a snorer may have periods of disturbed breathing during upper respiratory tract infection when the nose is blocked and the tonsils and adenoids are inflamed. In this situation, appropriate decongestant treatment and, when indicated, antibiotic treatment should be used first.

When obstructive sleep apnoea is severe and affecting the child's well-being (failure to thrive, heart failure or poor daytime function), the therapeutic options include surgery, nasal CPAP or bi-level CPAP (see below) and occasionally oral appliances.

Tonsillectomy or adeno-tonsillectomy is the first-choice treatment when enlarged tonsils and adenoids are present, as is often the case. Surgery is usually performed with the child as an *inpatient*. Although open to debate, young patients should be monitored carefully in the 24 hours following surgery for signs of complications that can be life-threatening. This is particularly so in children less than three years of age with disturbed breathing of more than ten apnoeas per hour and with low oxygen. The child may need to be monitored for apnoea, which may occur soon after surgery, and for post-operative haemorrhages. Because the severity of sleep apnoea is a risk factor for increased complication post-operatively, a sleep study to precisely define the number of apnoeas is usually required before surgery. Adeno-tonsillectomy, however, is not always successful and some children continue to snore and have apnoeas afterwards.

Nasal continuous airway pressure devices (nCPAP) and bi-level continuous pressure devices (bi-level CPAP) are used successfully in children. Sometimes they are used as a temporary measure before surgery; other times they are adopted for prolonged periods, such as when surgery has failed or is not possible. With bi-level CPAP the pressure increases when the child breathes in and decreases when they breathe out, and it is easier to tolerate than nasal CPAP. In nasal CPAP the airflow is continuous at the same pressure throughout the breathing cycle.

The above discussion highlights the uncertainty surrounding treatment of obstructive sleep apnoea. Often, parents face the question: 'Should my child have an adeno-tonsillectomy, or should I wait?' It seems reasonable to say that if the child has sleep apnoea severe enough to cause failure to thrive, heart failure (when other causes are excluded) and difficulty with daytime function and schooling, then surgery should be considered. If the parents are concerned because of loud snoring and a few witnessed apnoeas, but the child is well, a wait-and-watch approach is a reasonable compromise. This decision is made more reassuring if an overnight sleep monitoring shows only minimal abnormalities.

❇ Bed wetting (nocturnal enuresis)

Bed wetting is very common and presents in 25–30 per cent of four- to five-year-old children. It declines with age but is still present in 3 per cent of twelve-year-olds. By convention, nocturnal enuresis is diagnosed as such if present after the age of five. A distinction is made between children who never manage to remain dry at night (primary enuresis), who represent more than 90 per cent of the cases, and children who after a few months of being dry start bed wetting again (secondary enuresis).

It should be emphasised that before a diagnosis of nocturnal enuresis is made, a careful examination must exclude conditions that can cause bed wetting. Specifically, urinary tract infection, bladder or kidney abnormalities, and other more rare neurological conditions may cause enuresis. Diabetes should also be excluded as a cause of nocturnal bed wetting in a child. These medical conditions, and sometimes psychological problems such as the birth of a new child or conflict with the parents, are the usual causes of secondary enuresis.

Primary enuresis, on the other hand, is thought to be due to maturational delay in both capacity to concentrate urine and bladder control during sleep. Genetic factors are also present, because parents of children who wet their bed have frequently been bed wetters themselves. In fact, if both parents had enuresis during childhood, in 75 per cent of cases their children are also enuretic. Bed wetting can occur in all stages of sleep but predominantly in non-REM sleep.

Primary enuresis does not result in any physical complication. However, it can be quite testing for the child and parents. The child may be bullied at school, or may refuse to go on excursions or camps so as to avoid being embarrassed in front of other children.

Lack of understanding of the problem on the parents' part may lead to unorthodox remedies that may be harmful. The child may be punished or their penis or urethra manipulated, causing physical injury.

Treatment

The child will eventually reach bladder control as they get older. When intervention is needed, the pad and bell alarm system and pharmacological intervention can be used.

The alarm system is considered the most successful type of intervention. The pad is attached to the underwear and contains a switch that closes with moisture, triggering an alarm.

The sound goes off as soon as the child starts wetting. Initially the child may not wake at all, in which case the parents are encouraged to try and wake them up and take them to the bathroom. Eventually the child starts waking with the alarm and finishes urinating in the toilet. Dry nights will start alternating with wet ones until the child remains dry. The process may take four to eight weeks and is successful in 70 per cent of cases. Relapse when the alarm is discontinued can occur in up to 40 per cent of cases.

The medication most commonly used for many years was Imipramine (a tricyclic antidepressant), 25–50 milligrams of which was given at bedtime. It is effective while the child is on it, but enuresis recurs when ceased. Imipramine affects sleep structure, can cause a dry mouth, excessive sweating and other side-effects, and is currently not recommended.

At present, Desmopressin (Minirin Nasal Spray™), a hormone that retains fluid and concentrates urine, is the medication more commonly prescribed.

It is applied as one or two nasal sprays at bedtime. It is less effective in providing a permanent cure when compared with the pad and bell system and is not effective in every child. It can, however, be used when the child is away from home such as when camping or on holidays.

✳ Sleepiness and tiredness in children and adolescents

Most of what was said in Chapter 6 about sleepiness and tiredness applies to children as well. However, some aspects more specific to childhood are worth considering here.

Young children do not complain of sleepiness, and the problem does not usually come to the parents' attention until school age. Teachers may recognise difficulty with learning, poor concentration, reluctance to participate in classroom activities or napping at school. The degree of the problem can vary and need not necessarily be severe. A child who falls asleep daily at school is more likely to be recognised as sleepy than one in whom the problem manifests with poor concentration and distractibility.

The child may be fidgety, talkative, disruptive and move around excessively. The range of symptoms overlaps with attention deficit hyperactivity disorder (ADHD). The relation between ADHD and disturbance of sleep–wake function has not been studied, but it is a clinical observation that adults with narcolepsy or non-REM narcolepsy often have children diagnosed with ADHD. Stimulants are used for both conditions and are effective.

Adolescents constitute an important group in whom complaints of fatigue and sleepiness are common. *Fatigue* appears to be the preferred word even when sleepiness is the underlying problem. The adolescent appears to be more sleepy because of an intrinsic increase in sleepiness at puberty and because of a reduction in the quantity of sleep obtained. Sleep requirement remains high in puberty (nine hours on average), but sleep needs are often not met because of social expectations and peer pressure. The use of recreational drugs also becomes an issue at this age. How these factors affect performance varies with each individual.

Symptoms of *narcoleptic syndromes* frequently start at this age. However, the diagnosis of narcolepsy (see Chapter 6) or non-REM narcolepsy (idiopathic hypersomnolence) may be difficult because not all symptoms may be present at once. For example, the adolescent may be sleepy without having irresistible sleep attacks. Sleepiness may be the only symptom, without hypnagogic hallucinations, sleep paralysis or cataplexy. It is even more difficult if the child has only hypnagogic (at the beginning of sleep) or hypnopompic (at the end of sleep) hallucinations, because these may be interpreted as symptoms of psychiatric illness such as schizophrenia. If the only symptom is cataplexy (lack of muscle power during laughing, anger or frustration), it may be mistaken for anxiety disorder or conversion syndrome (hysteria).

More recently (see Chapter 6), some young people with increased sleepiness tendency and complaining of tiredness have been labelled as having chronic fatigue syndrome. The end-result of this set of circumstances is that often the diagnosis is missed for years, with severe consequences for the young person in terms of schooling and personal development. Treatment with stimulant medications is usually effective (see Chapters 6 and 8).

A particular form of overt sleepiness goes under the name of *Kleine-Levin syndrome*. In this condition there is a sudden or subacute onset of sleepiness in children between the age of twelve and eighteen. In the initial description, compulsive eating was also present. Children with this syndrome may put themselves to bed and can sleep up to twenty hours a day. They may wake up during the day to void and for binge eating. They can be found in the middle of the night in the kitchen where they eat anything they can get hold of. At times they may appear irritable and profusely sweaty. The attack may last from one day to a few weeks and re-occur after a few months. There is normal behaviour in between attacks. No consistent abnormalities have been found. A viral illness precedes the onset of the syndrome in approximately 50 per cent of cases.

Kleine-Levin syndrome is more common in males than females. At times, the attacks may present only with sleepiness without overeating.

Treatment includes the use of stimulants during the sleepiness episode. The condition tends to improve spontaneously over time. Careful medical examination is needed to exclude brain pathology, which may present in a similar manner.

8

Medications and sleep

- Many medications used for other medical conditions can affect sleep and wake function, causing sleepiness or insomnia.
- Alcohol, caffeine and nicotine cause poor sleep quality, both on their own and in combination.
- Sleeping tablets and stimulant medications are useful in specific sleep and wake disorders, and safe when used under supervision.
- Melatonin is classified as a 'natural substance' and does not go through the same strict scrutiny as other prescription medications. It should be used with caution because its long-term effects are not yet known.

There are many substances, both prescription and non-prescription, that can affect sleep. Some are used for 'recreational' purposes, others are prescribed to try and improve sleep and wake, and many more are used to treat other medical conditions.

✳ Non-prescription substances

Non-prescription substances that may be used routinely, and that affect sleep, include coffee, caffeine and alcohol.

Table 8.1 Caffeine content of various items (in mg)

Cup of coffee	90–150
Decaf-drink	2–4
Tea	30–70
Cola drinks	15–30
Chocolate bar	30–40
NO DOZ™	100
DYNAMO tablets™	100
ERGODRYL™	100
CAFERGOT™	100

Caffeine

Caffeine is contained in a variety of beverages and also as part of medications (Table 8.1). Caffeine has a stimulatory effect which starts about twenty to thirty minutes after ingestion and lasts for a few hours. Caffeine can also be found in tablet form as an over-the-counter preparation. Truck drivers and army personnel use it to increase alertness. The dose varies from 200 to 600 milligrams. Five cups of strong coffee are roughly equivalent to one 5 milligram tablet of dexamphetamine. There is variability from one person to another in the response to caffeine, but if taken in the evening it can interfere with sleep. It takes longer to fall asleep, and sleep structure is altered with reduction of slow wave sleep (deep sleep). The combination of alcohol, coffee and nicotine is particularly disruptive.

Alcohol

Alcohol has many actions among which is sedation. If a person has had more than two or three drinks in the evening before going to bed, sleep onset is faster but the quality of sleep is poor in the second part of the night. The sedative effect of alcohol wears off after two to three hours and it is followed by a rebound of alertness, which causes sleep to be very light. Sometimes it causes recurrent awakenings through the night. In chronic alcoholics, sleep is very fragmented causing severe sleep deprivation.

Snoring and sleep apnoeas will worsen if the person drinks alcohol before going to sleep, as the muscle relaxant effect of alcohol causes the muscles in the back of the throat to become floppier, making them more likely to vibrate and collapse.

❋ Medications used in other medical conditions

Most of the medications we use have side-effects. Sleep disturbances, both insomnia and sleepiness, are common. However, some groups of medications are known to alter sleep in a consistent way.

Betablockers

These are commonly used for the management of high blood pressure, angina (coronary artery disease), and for prophylaxis and prevention of migraine. There are different types of betablockers with different side-effects. Daytime tiredness/sleepiness and nightmares are particularly common.

Other anti-hypertensive medications

Other medications used to control blood pressure, such as prazosin (Minipress™, Pressin™), methyldopa (Aldomet™), and clonidine (Catapres™), can cause sedation during the day and also alter sleep structure.

Anticonvulsants

All medications used for epilepsy can cause daytime sedation and affect quality of sleep.

Antidepressants

All antidepressants affect daytime function as well as sleep. Both the 'old' group, such as amitriptyline (Tryptanol™), nor-triptyline (Allegron™), desipramine (Pertofran™), trimipramine (Surmontil™), doxepin (Deptran™) and mianserin (Tolvon™), and the 'new' group such as fluoxetine (Prozac™), paroxetine (Aropax™) and sertraline (Zoloft™), are strong REM suppressants and cause changes in sleep structure. The 'old' group promotes sleepiness and are used at night as sleeping tablets. However, the effect often spills into the day, causing daytime drowsiness and other side-effects (see below). The 'new' group, on the other hand, tends to have a stimulatory effect and can cause insomnia.

✳ Sleeping tablets

As discussed in Chapter 5, sleeping tablets are sometimes used for a brief period to help a person adjust to a stressful situation. They *do not cure the problem* but may be helpful at times.

The *ideal* sleeping tablet should:

- help in falling asleep quickly (within thirty minutes);
- not interfere with sleep structure; and
- not have any residual effect during the day.

Such a medication simply does not exist.

Table 8.2   Benzodiazepines: usual doses used to promote sleep in mg

Valium™	2–10
Serapax™	15–30
Murelax™	15–30
Normison™	10
Temaze™	10
Euhypnos™	10
Mogadon™	5
Halcion™	0.125
Rohypnol™	2

Barbiturates are no longer used since the advent of benzodiazepines (the Valium™ group). Benzodiazepines are the most commonly used sleeping tablets (Table 8.2).

Short-acting sleeping tablets are appropriate because they have less residual effect during the day. However, some individuals using the very short acting sleeping tablets such as triazolam (Halcion™) may develop some degree of anxiety during the day, and in the elderly confusion has been reported. A new group of short-acting *non*-benzodiazepine sleeping tablets are available which are said to have less risk of withdrawal symptoms. These include zopiclone (Imovane™, recommended dose 7.5 mg, a full tablet, or 3.25 mg, half tablet for the elderly) and zolpidem (not available in Australia).

Long-acting sleeping tablets are more suited in people with anxiety disorders, because the long action of the medication spills over into the day, reducing anxiety symptoms.

Continuous long-term use of benzodiazepine is not recommended. Usually, sleep onset is faster while using sleeping tablets and the length of sleep is slightly prolonged (by about thirty minutes). However, these effects tend to disappear after three to four weeks of daily use. Despite the fact that the effects of sleeping tablets tend to disappear after a few weeks, some patients need to continue taking the medication. One possible explanation for this is that the medication changed the 'perception' of sleep. That is, the patient *perceives* or *thinks* they have slept better. Also, in some people sleeping tablets can cause withdrawal symptoms after three to four weeks of continuous use if the medication is stopped abruptly. In particular, there can be worsening of insomnia and occasionally this may be more severe than before using the medication. The patient may also experience a more fragmented night, muscular aches and pains, and there can be confusion in the elderly. These symptoms can last from a few days to weeks and on rare occasions up to a year.

The short-acting sleeping tablet zopiclone (Imovane™) is said not to cause withdrawal symptoms.

Antidepressants as sleeping tablets

Antidepressants such as amitriptyline (Tryptanol™ and Endep™) and doxepin (Deptran™) have been used as sleeping tablets in people in whom insomnia was thought to be due to depressive illness. Doses of between 10 and 75 milligrams have been used for this purpose. However, the medication often tends to cause drowsiness during the day and with an increasing dose other symptoms may become troublesome, such as dry mouth, constipation, blurring of vision, excessive sweating, tremor, fast heart rate, and a sour or metallic taste in the mouth.

✳ Melatonin

Melatonin is a hormone produced within the brain by a structure called the pineal gland and regulated by the night and light cycle (see Figure 2 in Chapter 1). The level of melatonin increases during darkness and decreases during daylight. When the level has increased, it signals the body the optimal time to start sleep. Melatonin can thus be considered a 'sleep-promoting' substance rather than a sleeping tablet as such.

Melatonin has been claimed to have many properties, from modulation of the immune system and an anti-tumour effect, to an anti-stress and anti-depression action. The level of melatonin (the 'sleep hormone') decreases with age and it has been suggested that this is responsible for poor sleep quality in the elderly.

Because of the many claims for melatonin and the fact that it is a 'natural substance', it has great appeal and has been used by millions of people around the world. However, melatonin is not a prescription substance and so does not go through the rigorous scrutiny prescription medications go through in terms of both dosage and formulation. A wide range of doses have been used, from a few milligrams up to 100 or more milligrams. It is not clear what potential side-effects the use of melatonin may cause—in particular, long-term side-effects.

In the past, the use of some other 'natural products' turned out not to be safe. For example, the use of some formulation of tryptophane (another natural substance used to promote sleep and in vogue a few years ago) caused severe muscular disease and, in a few cases, death.

Our current knowledge allows us to make the following points regarding melatonin:

- Doses of between 0.1 and 0.3 milligrams achieve levels in the blood similar to physiological body production.
- Doses above 5 milligrams are unlikely to give any extra beneficial effect.

So far, melatonin has been used in two ways: as a 'synchroniser', and as a sleeping tablet. A typical example of the synchroniser effect is found in people with delayed sleep phase syndrome (see Chapter 5), where the set point to fall asleep is delayed past midnight. In this situation the use of melatonin early in the evening, at 6–7 p.m., may help in resetting sleep to an earlier time with a shift of thirty to sixty minutes per day of treatment.

However, melatonin appears also to have a mild 'sleeping tablet' property, increasing the tendency to fall asleep about thirty minutes to an hour after ingestion. It does not appear to alter sleep structure, nor to cause a hangover effect the next day. Both actions—as synchroniser and as sleeping tablet—are considered useful to counteract jet lag symptoms by taking melatonin (0.3–5 milligrams) at bedtime in the new time zone. However, for jet lag the synchronising effect of exposure to light is more powerful than melatonin. On theoretical grounds, the combination of 'light' therapy and melatonin may have an added effect.

Side-effects of melatonin

No significant side-effects have been reported so far, but the long-term use of melatonin could have potential side-effects.

Animal studies suggest that melatonin has a modulation action on the production of antibodies by binding to immune system cells. Potential interaction with sex hormones has also been reported in animals, such as testicular and ovary atrophy (diminuition in size and function) in hamsters. At present, it is unclear what doses are safe in children, if any. For the above reasons, at least long-term use of melatonin cannot be recommended.

✻ Stimulant medications

There are two stimulant medications available in Australia, dexamphetamine and methylphenidate (Ritalin™). In both cases, an authority from the Department of Health in each state is needed for a prescription. The medications are used for the treatment of narcolepsy and other forms of hypersomnolence and in attention deficit disorders.

Dexamphetamine can be prescribed under the PBS (Pharmaceutical Benefits Scheme) and part of the cost is covered by Medicare. The cost of Ritalin™ must be entirely paid by the patient.

The action of the two drugs is similar, but some individuals respond better to one or the other. Both medications work by increasing the level of nor-adrenaline and dopamine in the brain, increasing alertness.

Starting treatment with stimulant medications

Treatment is started and continued under medical supervision and advice. The usual starting dose is half to one tablet

(2.5–5 milligrams of dexamphetamine, or 5–10 milligrams of Ritalin™) at breakfast and half to one tablet at midday. The dose is then slowly increased according to how the person responds.

Some patients take the entire daily dose at breakfast; others spread them through the day. The use of medication late in the afternoon, after 4–5 p.m., is discouraged because it can interfere with sleep onset and sleep quality. Once an effective dose is found, the medication does not need to be used continuously. Some people use it only when they drive, others during working days but not on weekends, while others use it every day.

Possible side-effects of stimulant medications

Reported side-effects include headaches, irritability, nervousness and tremor, lack of appetite, insomnia, palpitations and gastrointestinal complaints. Side-effects such as lack of appetite, insomnia and weight loss are usually transient. Tics (twitches) can occur, particularly in children. Dryness of the mouth, constipation, nausea and an unpleasant taste are also reported on occasion. On very rare occasions, a *paradoxical effect* is noted. It seems that thirty to sixty minutes after taking the medication the person experiences an increase in sleepiness. The reason is not known.

There is little evidence suggesting that stimulant medications can cause an increase in blood pressure at the dose normally used. However, in combination with certain new anti-depressants—for example, venlafaxine—an increase in blood pressure is sometimes seen.

All stimulant medications tend to reduce appetite, and in *diabetic people* this may result in reduction of food intake which requires adjustment of insulin or oral medication.

Stimulant medication and pregnancy

The potential for side-effects to the foetus is not well established and it is recommended that women who are planning to fall pregnant should not use the medication.

Stimulant medication and breastfeeding

The breast milk of nursing mothers contains a higher concentration of stimulant medication than the mother's blood. Therefore, nursing mothers who have narcolepsy should consider reducing the dose of stimulant medication to maintain their wakefulness, but caution is urged.

Stimulant medication and psychiatric illness

Stimulant medication can cause hallucinations and altered mental states, particularly at high dosages and in people with a pre-existing psychiatric illness. The stimulants used in therapeutic doses do not appear to affect emotional stability.

Stimulant medication and cardiovascular complications

The occurrence of cardiovascular complications (such as strokes and heart failure) is rarely reported in people using stimulant medications for medical purposes. In the cases reported, the dose has been 100 milligrams of dexamphetamine and 200 milligrams of methylphenidate per day for several years. Heart failure has been reported in people injecting stimulants intravenously for recreational purpose.

Tolerance to stimulant medication

Tolerance refers to the need to increase the dose of the stimulant to maintain the same level of alertness. At the dose that we normally use, tolerance is not seen. However, it appears that the higher the dose of the medication, the more likely that tolerance may develop at some stage. Intermittent use of the medication has been suggested as a useful strategy to diminish the potential development of tolerance (for example, stopping the medication at weekends). However, there is no evidence for this recommendation and it may cause unnecessary hardship to the patient.

Drug dependency (drug addiction)

Stimulant medication has a high abuse potential and can produce dependence. However, most users do not become addicted to the drug. In particular, when the medication is taken for medical purposes (and *not* for recreation) and under medical supervision, the potential for dependency is reduced.

✳ Modafinil

Modafinil (Modiadol™, Provigil™) is a new stimulant medication developed by the French pharmaceutical company La Fon. It is currently used in the United States and Europe for the treatment of narcolepsy and non-REM narcolepsy (idiopathic hypersomnolence). It is not marketed in Australia even though patients can import the medication for individual use.

Modafinil is a non-amphetamine stimulant which increases wakefulness. It has a different mechanism to that of dexamphetamine and methylphenidate (Ritalin™). Data in animals suggests that modafinil action is more selectively targeted to the thalamus (a deep structure in the brain important for sleep and wakefulness). The alerting effect of modafinil is similar in intensity to dexamphetamine and Ritalin™, but side-effects are less common.

In a trial comparing modafinil with a placebo (a dummy tablet) in 283 narcoleptic patients, headache was more common among subjects using modafinil. Although individual patients may experience anxiety and restlessness, as with amphetamines, on average increased anxiety was not more common than when a placebo was used. Modafinil is less likely to cause withdrawal symptoms and dependence compared to amphetamines.

The dose of modafinil varies from 200–400 milligrams per day, usually in two divided doses. As with other stimulant medications, the use of modafinil should be avoided if pregnancy is planned. It should also be noted that the use of modafinil may reduce the effectiveness of oral contraceptives.

9

Sleep disorders and driving

- Sleep apnoea, narcolepsy and chronic sleep deprivation carry an increased risk of motor vehicle accidents.
- Sleep deprivation and young adults are a dangerous combination.
- Driving while sleep-deprived may have the same risk as driving under the influence of alcohol.
- Under current regulations, people who suffer from sleep apnoea or narcolepsy cannot drive unless they are under-going treatment.

✳ Sleep deprivation and car accidents

It is increasingly recognised that fatigue is often a contributing factor in motor vehicle accidents even though it is difficult to demonstrate or document that a driver has fallen asleep at the wheel. However, when information is available it can be shown that car accidents are more likely when sleep deprivation is present. For example, accidents are more likely at night between midnight and 6 a.m., the longer the hours of driving, and the lesser the amount of sleep in the previous 24 hours.

There are many reasons for increased daytime sleepiness, including:

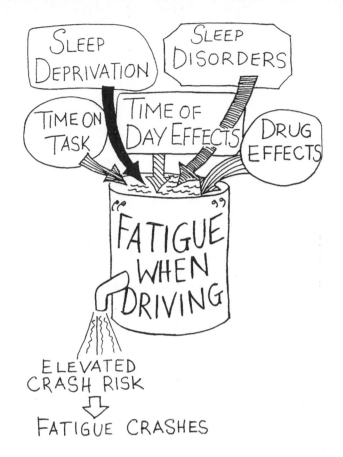

Figure 21 Causes of fatigue/sleepiness while driving

1 sleep deprivation due to:
- shift working; or
- prolonged sleep restriction;
2 fragmentation of sleep due to sleep disorders such as sleep apnoea, periodic limb movement disorder, narcoleptic syndrome;
3 time of the day; and
4 use of medications.

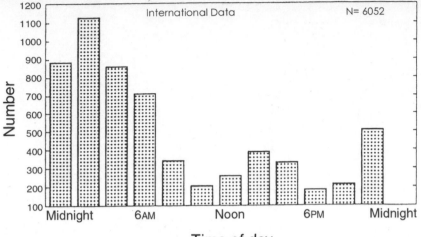

Figure 22 Number of motor vehicle accidents at various times of the day (Republished with permission of the American Sleep Disorders Association, 'Catastrophes, sleep and public policy: consensus report' M. Mitler, M. Carskadon et al., *Sleep*, vol. 11)

The early hours of the morning between midnight and 6 a.m. are the most critical period of the day for motor vehicle accidents, followed by early afternoon (Figure 22).

As mentioned in Chapter 6, shift working always causes sleep debts. This is dangerous for night workers who sometimes sacrifice daytime hours of rest for social commitments or for other jobs.

Perhaps the most common cause of chronic tiredness and fatigue is restriction of hours of rest dictated by long hours at work, commuting time and social pressures. This is a particular problem in teenagers and young adults.

Figure 23 illustrates the number of serious accidents in New South Wales in 1993. It can be seen that the highest percentage is accounted for the age between the teens and early adulthood, indicating that young age is a very powerful predictor and a

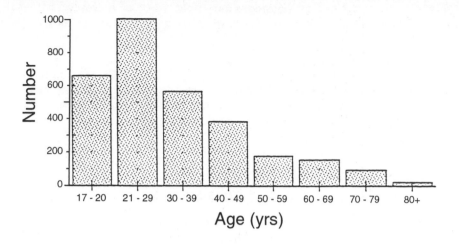

Figure 23   Effect of age in fatigue related car accidents

risk factor for serious accidents. This is likely a result of the fact that young people are more likely to drive long hours and to become sleep-deprived because of work and social engagements.

✳ Sleep apnoea, narcolepsy and car accidents

Studies conducted in both sleep disorders centres as well as in the community consistently suggest that patients with sleep apnoea are three to seven times more likely to have a motor vehicle accident. However, the absolute number is small and, as shown in Figure 23, young age is a much higher risk factor.

It is suggested that patients with narcolepsy have a high risk of falling asleep while driving, as well as of exposing themselves to work-related accidents.

The importance of obstructive sleep apnoea and narcolepsy is recognised by the Road Traffic Authority, which has set strict

Table 9.1   Restrictions on holding a car, light truck or motorcycle licence for people with sleep disorders (Reprinted with permission of Austroads)

Narcolepsy	All patients suspected of having narcolepsy should be warned about potential impact on road safety.
	High-risk patients should not drive until disorder investigated and treated effectively. High risk includes severe daytime sleepiness, uncontrolled cataplexy, or history of motor vehicle crashes caused by inattention or sleepiness.
	High-risk individuals whose condition is not amenable to treatment within two months or are unwilling to accept treatment or unwilling to restrict driving on advice should not drive.
	All cases of narcolepsy should be subject to review at least annually. Initial sleep physician or neurologist opinion recommended.
	Where the patient has been involved in a crash as a result of sleeping at the wheel, driving should be disallowed until the condition has been successfully treated.
Sleep Apnoea	All patients suspected of having sleep apnoea should be warned about potential impact on road safety.
	High-risk patients should not drive until disorder investigated and treated effectively. High risk includes severe daytime sleepiness or history of motor vehicle crashes caused by inattention or sleepiness.
	High-risk individuals whose condition is not amenable to treatment within two months or are unwilling to accept treatment or unwilling to restrict driving on advice should not drive.
	High-risk patients with proven sleep apnoea should be reviewed annually by a sleep physician.
	Where the patient has been involved in a crash as a result of sleeping at the wheel, driving should be disallowed until the condition has been successfully treated.

Patients should be made aware about the effects of their condition on driving and advised of their legal obligation to notify the Driver Licensing Authority where driving is likely to be affected. As a last resort, practitioners may themselves advise the Driver Licensing Authority.

regulations for certification for fitness to hold a driver's licence (see Table 9.1).

For driver's licence category A, it is required that persons with either sleep apnoea or narcolepsy be undergoing treatment to be allowed to drive.

For a commercial driver's licence, a diagnosis of narcolepsy virtually excludes the possibility of holding a licence. These

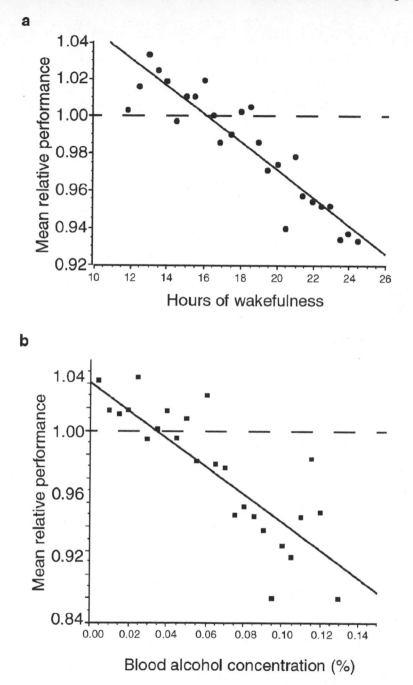

Figure 24 **Effect of sleep deprivation (hours of wakefulness) and alcohol on performance (Reprinted by permission of *Nature*, D. Dawson & K Reid 'Fatigue, alcohol and performance impairment', 1997 Macmillan Magazine Ltd)**

regulations are currently being revised to allow for individual differences and degree of severity in sleepiness tendency.

It is surprising that such strict regulations are applied to the category of obstructive sleep apnoea and narcolepsy but no restrictions are imposed on shift workers. Neurophysiological testing has shown that the drop in performance of sleep-deprived people can be compared to a person with an increased level of alcohol.

Figure 24 shows that there is a progressive drop in performance with sleep deprivation. After 22 hours of wakefulness, the decrease in performance is similar to a person with a blood level of 0.1 (the legal limit being 0.05). The tests used did not involve driving, but it can be suggested that driving while sleep-deprived may carry a similar risk as driving when intoxicated by alcohol.

10

Dreams and dreaming

- Dreaming is awareness of mental activity during sleep.
- Dreams are what we remember of dreaming when we wake up.
- Because memory is not very active during sleep, recollection of dreams is often not precise and details are easily forgotten.
- Everyone dreams, though some people never remember dreaming.
- The content of dreams is mostly *internally* generated and is little influenced by external sensations.
- Dreaming is a vehicle to our inner world, but its language requires introspection to be fully understood.
- Only the dreamer can 'interpret' their dreams.

✳ Dreams in history

Dreaming and dreams are fundamental experiences of human life and their importance can be traced back through the ages. In antiquity, dreams were considered to be messengers from the gods. They were perceived as supernatural and, as such, were thought to be predictive of the future and as having healing powers. Hippocrates the Ancient Greek physician who is considered to be the 'father of medicine', used dreams to diagnose bodily ailments. In Egypt and Greece, temples were built for people to evoke dreams to obtain guidance for the future and medical cures.

In Greek and Roman literature, dreams are also divine and prophetic. It is in a dream that Aeneas was told by Hector to leave Troy and to found a new city, which eventually became Rome. Julius Caesar's wife dreamt of his assassination in the Senate. In the Middle Ages the prophetic interpretation of dreams persisted, despite their also being considered a reflection of evil, in keeping with the culture of the time. Saint Francis abandoned the wealth of his family and started the Franciscan brotherhood following a dream in which Jesus Christ talked to him.

In more recent times, as human thinking moved towards a more man-centred world and the rational mind started to prevail over the religious one, dreams have been, at times, considered insignificant and without meaning because of their frequent 'non-rational' nature. Eventually, Sigmund Freud's efforts to apply scientific methods to the analysis of the mind established dreaming as an important mental process, irrespective of the controversy surrounding his interpretation of dreams.

In our everyday life the wide interest in dreams is driven more by the fact that they are perceived as positive, allusive and mystical than by the less frequent negative experience, such as nightmares and anxiety dreams.

The positive connotation of dreams is reflected in many languages by sayings such as 'it's a dream come true', 'it could only happen in my dreams' and 'the stuff dreams are made of'. There is, in fact, an entire nation built on a dream, the 'American dream'. This was eventually shaken and questioned in 1963 in an emotional speech by Dr Martin Luther King, who spelled out the aspirations of a black nation using the famous line, 'I have a dream that one day . . .' King gave his dream a powerful sense of destiny and inevitability and, at least in this case, it has come true.

Controversy persists over what dreams are, what they mean and how they should be interpreted, if at all. The following paragraphs are an attempt to justify the view that dreams are a vehicle to our inner world, drawing attention to ideas, feelings and attitudes that are part of our personality and which our *waking minds* may have overlooked or underestimated. By the same token, because our inner mind is influenced by the outside world, dreams can also highlight events that we have failed to notice during the day.

✳ What are dreaming and dreams?

Dreaming is the awareness of mental activity during sleep, which we report as dreams when awake. It testifies to the fact that sleep is an active process and not just the suspension of mental and bodily functions. Dreaming is a form of thinking and therefore is of great interest.

The key words in the above are *awareness, mental activity, sleep* and *awake*.

We will now look at how these four elements interact in the origin of dreaming and dreams.

Everyone dreams, and dreaming is not confined to REM sleep

It is now accepted that dreams and dreaming are not confined to REM sleep, but occur with similar frequency in non-REM sleep. However, there remains significant controversy surrounding this view, so it may be useful to review how our understanding has evolved over time.

For a long time the study of mental processes, including dreams, was negatively influenced by René Descartes' view that the body and the mind are separate entities, the former being measurable and the latter unmeasurable.

However, over the last 100 years our ability to measure physiological parameters, such as brain waves, and to correlate these measurements with specific mental functions, has proven this division of body and mind untenable.

As far as dreaming is concerned, the 1950s constituted ten years of major advances thanks to North American and European researchers. In 1892, George Trumbull Ladd had made the observation that the eyes move during sleep, following the images of dreams. However, it was not until 1953 that Eugene Aserinski, who was working with Nathaniel Kleitman in Chicago, observed rapid eye movements in sleeping infants and soon after the same observation could be made in adults. They also developed the methodology to record these eye movements on paper using small electrodes placed just above and lateral to the eyes. This ability to monitor the brain activity (EEG), eye movements and muscle tones allowed the description of what is now known as REM and non-

REM sleep. It was also noted that the eye movements were synchronous, and that the pulse rate and breathing became faster and more irregular, as if the body was in a state of activation. It was hypothesised that the sleeping person was moving their eyes in a purposeful manner, like someone following a scene. The step towards thinking that during REM the sleeping person was dreaming was made very quickly. This hypothesis was tested by waking the person during REM and asking whether they had been dreaming. The results were impressive, showing vivid dreams in 80 per cent of the awakenings from REM compared to 7 per cent in non-REM.

These observations were of great importance, even though they were not completely correct (see below). They demonstrated that dreaming (a mental activity, a process of the mind) was clearly linked to a measurable biological brain activity (a body process). They contradicted the diffusely held view that dreaming was a random, non-predictable experience. As we have seen in Chapter 1, REM sleep is cyclical, recurring four to five times a night.

Now researchers had a way to study dreams, because they could predict when the person was dreaming. Many questions could be answered. For example, people who stated that they never dream could be shown to be dreaming if woken during REM sleep. Dreaming is a biological function present in everybody, even though dream recall may vary from one person to another.

Similarly, the idea that people dream mostly in black and white, rather than in colour, was shown to be incorrect. If the person is questioned immediately after arousal, dreams are reported in colour, like waking experiences.

The popular belief that illnesses and certain foods can cause a person to dream more can also be explained simply by the fact that when people are unwell, they are more likely to wake up and therefore dream recall is increased.

Although the discovery of REM sleep has advanced enormously our understanding of dreaming and sleep, subsequent research started to question the view that REM sleep *equalled* dreaming. It became clear that the low percentage of dream recall in non-REM was due to the kind of question the person was asked on awakening. If *any mental activity* was considered—for example, thinking rather than just images—then dream recall in non-REM was found in up to 74 per cent of cases, not much different from 80 per cent in REM. It should be kept in mind that a major problem in the study of dreams and dreaming remains the fact that the person is awake when they report their dream, and therefore memory is a major determinant and variable from one individual to another.

In summary, it can be said that dreaming occurs both during REM and non-REM sleep and is a biological function present in everybody. Everybody dreams.

Self-awareness (consciousness), wakefulness, sleep and the process of dreaming

As mentioned previously, dreaming is awareness of mental activity during sleep. It is useful to consider aspects of awareness of mental activity during *wakefulness* to understand dreaming.

Wakefulness mental activity is heavily constrained by three elements: interaction with the outside world, the notion of time, and causality. I would argue that these three elements do not constrain mental activity during sleep and this is likely to explain the often bizarre and 'non-rational' nature of dreams (the activity of the dreaming mind) when reported by the waking mind.

During wakefulness there is full activation of sensory modalities, with literally millions of pieces of information being processed by the brain. This flooding of external stimuli allows us to interact with the external world within the complexity of human behaviour, which requires integration of sensory input and motor activity, modulated by previous experiences and emotional responses (feelings). Memory is central to this activity, as well as to a continuous learning process.

However, only a fraction of this complex processing work reaches awareness. This fact is well exemplified by the experience of *daydreaming*.

It is common to see people in their car, on their own, who are talking and moving their hands as if they are having an animated discussion. They are performing a complex task such as driving, but their 'mind' is elsewhere. They eventually find themselves a few kilometres down the road without full recollection of having driven that far. It is also common for students to be seated with a proper posture and looking at the teacher talking but focusing their awareness far from the classroom. Daydreaming is *internally generated* and mostly not influenced by external activity, at least until someone regains the daydreamer's attention!

During wakefulness, memory processes are involved both in information retrieval and acquisition of new information through the continuous sensory input and processing (learning). During sleep, however, memory has very little involvement in learning, because the external input process has shut down, although not completely. An example of this is the observation that the precise moment a person falls asleep cannot be remembered because it is not registered. In fact, the belief that we can learn during sleep ('sleep learning') is unproven.

During dreaming, information is stored in the short-term memory but does not proceed to permanent storage unless the person wakes up during the dream and starts thinking about its content. Unless this happens, the content of the dream will be rapidly forgotten. In fact, the best practice is to write it down immediately.

The sleeping mind also differs from the waking mind with regard to the role that time plays in its organisation. Time is fundamental to how the waking mind stores and retrieves information. Not so for the sleeping mind. Consider the following example. Imagine the situation where you bump your shin against a chair, causing intense pain in your leg. Your mind will record the experience as the *action* of hitting your shin against the chair, *causing* (followed by) the pain. We will memorise the action and the feeling associated with it as a temporal sequence (causality). Now imagine the situation where your mind recalls the events, but the time element is removed— that is, *first* hitting the chair and *then* the pain. Imagine retrieving the pain first, followed by retrieving hitting the chair. It would be bizarre and incomprehensible, 'unreal'. In fact, if your leg is hurting but you cannot remember having bumped it, the first reaction is: 'I must have hit something, but I can't remember doing so.' If the pain persists and the cause is not obvious, you will become concerned that something obscure or sinister has happened until an explanation is found.

I would argue that the *sleeping mind* operates mostly on internally generated information and that, in the organisation of dream content, time plays a less important role than for the waking mind.

During dreaming, thoughts, feelings and emotions, and their integration and interactions, are expressed through sequences of images. If we remember that dreams are the reporting by the *awake person* of what they remembered of dreaming, it is not surprising that they are often considered odd, irrational and difficult to follow.

An example of representing thoughts and emotions by means of images without temporal constraint, in a 'dream-like' fashion, can be found in the cinematic work of the French director Alain Resnais. In the late 1960s as a teenager I used to attend the projection of 'art films' at the local movie club, followed by a critical discussion and analysis. I still remember the film *Last Year At Marienbad*. This is the story of a year-long relationship between two lovers. The film sequences are organised not in a temporal progression over the twelve-month period, but are edited by association of thoughts and emotions conveyed through the use of images. The result was a sense of frustration for most of the audience, who could not understand what was going on. Only those film buffs who had read critical reviews in advance and knew what the director had intended could make any sense of the film. It obviously made sense to the director, Resnais, and it did have its own internal logic—but not to the uninformed members of the audience.

A similar situation may well happen with dreams. Because the material of dreaming is mostly internally retrieved, and interaction with the external world is reduced, images, thoughts and emotions are often processed with little regard to real time progression. This allows much more creativity to the mind. For example, the image of a place or a person and an emotion can be associated not within a temporal framework but because they share emotional similarity. This can be puzzling when the person recalls the dream after waking up. Nevertheless, it is a great source of information for the person who dreams the dream. Like in Resnais' film, it could be said that the dreamer is really the only one who can explain or 'interpret' the dream. This view would argue strongly against the belief that one's dreams can be interpreted by other people.

✳ The material dreams are made of

A lesson from children's dreams

The study of dreams in children of various ages provides great insight into the process of dreaming. A study of this nature is very difficult to perform. However, David Folkes and his team at the University of Wyoming, in the United States, managed to study a group of 'normal' children between the ages of three and ten over a period of five years. Each child was studied for nine consecutive nights each year for the five years. These researchers were able to gather information on children's dreams between the ages of three and fifteen years and on how their dreams changed over time. They found that dreaming and dream content follow a maturational process that parallels the stages of waking thought development.

In children aged from three to five, dreams are mostly static images drawn mostly from familiar surroundings and contain little social interaction. Animal images are often present.

Between the ages of five and seven, dreams become longer and the content contains more activity. Rather than simple images, the children are able to describe a setting for the dream events. The family members are often portrayed.

Between the ages of seven and nine the child starts to become aware of having thoughts and feelings within the dream. The content includes elements outside the family, such as friends and school environment. The dreams contain mostly a pleasant content.

From the age of ten through the mid-teen years, dreams become more complex and dynamic. Self-participation is more common. The content becomes less story-like, with abstract elements and thought-like activity becoming more prevalent.

In essence, this important and unique study demonstrated that dreaming is a dynamic process that follows the same maturational process as the waking mind. The source of dream material reflects the person's environmental experiences, cognitive maturation and social interactions. In this sense, it can be argued that dreaming may well have a learning function.

Another important observation made in this study is that when children were allowed to watch violent television programs the night before the investigation, their dreams did not have more aggressive, violent or antisocial content than following non-violent program viewing.

Dreams and recent events

Events that occurred in the immediate past are often found in dreams. Material that relates to the day before the dream, called *day residues*, is present in 35 per cent of dreams, according to the French researcher Michael Jouvet. He reported the analysis of 2525 of his own dreams. In 400 of them he recognised events that occurred within the previous fifteen days. The personality and recent emotional events seem to influence dream content. Some people appear to recall dreams easily, while others hardly ever do. Dreaming recall is increased during pregnancy. Negative feelings are more common in subjects who have recently divorced and have a depressed mood, compared to people in a stable relationship. Another interesting observation in this group is that their mood starts to improve when the image of the former spouse appears in their dreams. This could suggest an active role of dreaming in integrating recent traumatic events in the person's life.

Awareness of external sensations is reduced during dreaming but is not completely abolished. It is a common experience that when the alarm clock goes off in the morning and the person is dreaming, the sound may be incorporated in the dream as a telephone or a doorbell ringing, perhaps in an attempt to prolong sleep. Researchers have measured the effect of external stimulation on dreams. Dement and Wolpert applied sound, light and water spray to sleeping people during REM sleep and then woke them a few minutes later. They found that spraying water, a touching sensation, was more commonly incorporated in dreams than were light and sound. Another interesting finding in their study is that there was correspondence between the length of time the stimulation was applied and the length of the dream. This observation seems to put to rest another commonly held belief: that dreams, even when they are long, actually occur in a fraction of a second. This view became popular following a famous dream reported by Albert Maury. He dreamed of being ill in his bedroom at the time of the French Revolution and of witnessing frightful scenes of murder. He was brought in front of a tribunal and condemned to death by decapitation. When the guillotine fell, he felt his head separate from his body and woke in a state of extreme anxiety. He soon realised that the top of the bed had fallen over his neck. Maury reasoned that the dream must have started and finished in the fraction of time between the trauma and the awakening. Experiments like those of Dement and Wolpert make this interpretation unlikely.

As mentioned above, increased night awakening and sleep fragmentation because of medical illnesses may be associated with *increased awareness* of dreaming, and the person reports of *dreaming more*. However, it is said that patients with serious medical conditions such as cancer, severe heart failure or major depression have more negative dreams and dreams with death content. This finding can probably be explained simply by the influence of daytime thoughts and restriction in body function on their dreams.

Patients with narcolepsy report more vivid dreams in keeping with abnormal REM sleep. Again, this could be explained by the fact that narcoleptic subjects wake up more at night, as well as being sleepy during the day, thus increasing the chance of dream recall.

Medications such as benzodiazepines and antidepressants (see Chapter 8) reduce dream recall, because of their action of REM suppression. Alcohol also has the same effect. If these drugs are withdrawn, then there is a rebound of vivid dreams. This can be particularly disturbing with benzodiazepine and alcohol withdrawal. Other medications such as betablockers (used for high blood pressure, coronary artery disease and migraine) and L-dopa (used for Parkinson's disease and occasionally for periodic limb movement disorder) can increase the frequency of dreams and of nightmares.

Something special during REM sleep: 'lucid dreams'

Lucid dreams are dreams during which the dreamer is aware they are dreaming. It is like watching yourself in a dream. Reports of lucid dreams are not common, being between 1 and 2 per cent of dream memories. However, it is reported in up to 20 per cent of people who practise meditation regularly. For example, the person may be dreaming of flying, realise they are dreaming but decide to continue enjoying the sensation of being in the air. The dreamer can, in fact, manipulate the dream and interact with it.

This ability led to the demonstration that lucid dreams occur during REM sleep. The experiment was ingenuous. The researchers worked with people who had frequent lucid dreams and recorded their EEG (electroencephalogram) and eye movements. The dreamers were trained and instructed to communicate *from within the dream* by moving their eyes in a specific sequence when they were witnessing a dream (lucid dream). Each time they signalled a lucid dream they were actually in REM sleep. Lucid dreams are experienced as 'different' from other dreams. However, when their transcripts are analysed the only difference is that lucid dreams appear to have more body movement and more sound than non-lucid dreams.

Dreams in the blind

Blind people do dream, but studies in this population are limited. When blindness has been present from birth, no visual imagery is reported. If someone has become blind after a period of normal vision, the frequency of images in their dreams becomes progressively more rare the longer the period of blindness.

✳ Is there a specific dream centre?

Until recently we did not have the technology to help this line of research. The advent of positive emission tomography (PET), which can identify which parts of the brain are functionally active, should advance our understanding of the anatomy of dreaming.

Prior to PET, some researchers had hypothesised that dreaming requires 'global' brain activation, or at least the activity of a network of centres. Others claimed that the right side of the brain is predominantly responsible for dreaming. The non-dominant hemisphere (the right in right-handed people) is mostly involved with visual and spatial tasks. The dominant hemisphere (the left in right-handed people) is responsible for verbal, logical and analytical processing. The similarity of dream activity with right brain function led to the hypothesis that dreams are products of the right brain. It was pointed out that if dreams are a right-sided function, the information needs to be transferred to the left side for dreams to be reported after awakening (the left side in right-handed people is responsible for speech). However, it is known that some patients with severe epilepsy, in whom the right and left hemispheres have been separated surgically, can still dream and report dreaming. If the above hypothesis was correct, these people should be able to dream but be unable to report the content.

Some aspects of dreaming may also be due to poor communication between the right and left brain. Michael Jouvet analysed dreams in which there were both images and verbal messages. In 54 per cent of cases the dreamer could recall the content of the message but could not identify the messenger's face. In 13 per cent of cases the messenger could be recognised, but the message was incomprehensible. This led to the suggestion that the often bizarre nature of dreams may be due to poor coordination between the right hemisphere (responsible for face recognition) and the left (which is responsible for speech).

It should also be noted that in blind people, visual imagery becomes progressively more rare and may disappear entirely after forty to fity years of blindness. This suggests that the occipital cortex, in the back of the brain on both right and left sides, is involved in dreaming. Animal experiments also support this view.

It seems intuitive to say that there are many anatomical structures that interact during dreaming. Advances in brain imaging should clarify this question in the near future.

✳ Do dreams need to be interpreted?

The idea that dreams need interpretation implies that dreams have a hidden or secret meaning. Usually we hide from others information about ourselves that is too important, or that we don't want people to know or of which we are ashamed. This idea, legitimised by Freud's use of dreams as the 'royal road to the unconscious' and the psychoanalytic association of dreams with psychiatric illnesses, has encouraged a pathological view of dreams. Some of our dreaming may well reflect emotional problems but no more or no less than our daytime thoughts do. Some dreams may be recurrent and unsettling, as some of our thoughts are.

The use of 'symbols' in dreams does not imply an attempt by the mind to disguise their meaning, as is often assumed. Symbols are a part of our society and culture, and they are used in our language to communicate with each other. It is thus not surprising that symbols appear in our dreams. For example, we give flowers to someone to express our affection for them—red roses for passion, the olive branch for peace, or the four-leaf clover for good luck.

Each of us also has our own *personal* symbols. Consider the following example. It is reported by Plato that when Socrates was offered by Crito, one of his disciples, a safe passage to avoid the death penalty, he described to him the following dream. He had seen a beautiful woman dressed in white who had come to him and said: 'Oh Socrates, in three days from now you will go to Phtia.' Crito was surprised by the dream. However, the master observed that the dream was quite clear. The woman dressed in white was predicting his death. (Phtia was the world of the dead.) It should be noted that white was the colour of mourning and death in the ancient Greek and Roman cultures, as it is today among the Chinese. If Socrates had lived in our time and in certain societies, the woman would probably be dressed in black. The number 'three' also had a special meaning at that time, representing the three dimensions of time: past, present and future.

I have tried to demonstrate in this chapter that dreaming is a physiological function that integrates and complements mental activity during wakefulness. The experiences with children have shown that dreams are initially simple, often with a happy content. As the individual self evolves with more abstract thinking, interpersonal relationships and emotional interactions, the structure of our dreams becomes more composite and its language more sophisticated, including the use of symbols.

Given the primarily internal origin of dream material, if interpretation is needed, only the dreamer can determine what meaning to ascribe to it. Paying attention to our *own* dreams is what is needed.

It is common experience that, if we are reading about dreaming or if we are going through psychological counselling or psychotherapy, dream recall and awareness is increased (that is, we appear to dream more). To pay attention to our dreams means to allocate some time to introspection, something that is not encouraged in our society. Thinking of what we do and how we live, and being critical (in a constructive way) of our behaviour and our feelings, is time well spent. Exactly the same applies to our dreams, which by their own special nature allow us to explore ourselves from a different angle. Counsellors, psychologists, psychiatrists or other professionals are not needed to interpret our dreams. They can, however, help in training the person in how to look at their dreams. Consider the following example.

A woman was referred because of insomnia and disturbing dreams. She described two dreams, which had been recurring over a period of twelve to eighteen months.

In one dream, she feels very upset because her partner has left her for another woman. In the second dream, she is extremely frightened when she sees someone, whom she identifies with herself, with blood on her teeth. Soon after, she wakes up.

Given the fact that both dreams had started around the same time, I asked if anything important had happened within the last twelve to eighteen months. She was unable to recall anything significant. Her first dream would be enough to upset anybody, but why was it recurring? This simple dream contains three elements: a strong feeling of unhappiness, the person herself and her boyfriend. It appeared that she needed to think about these three factors. She denied that her boyfriend had left her for someone else. However, upon prompting she said that about two years previously *she* had left *him* for two months to go and live with someone else, a workmate. She hadn't told the boyfriend why she had left him, but she eventually did so when she resumed living with him.

Continuing on this stream of thought, she reflected on how her boyfriend loved her more than she loved him. The reason she gave for coming back after two months was because she was scared of being alone and would rather continue a relationship that was unsatisfactory than be alone. She reflected on how her boyfriend had used any opportunity to make her feel guilty about having betrayed his trust. So, in the case of the first dream, the elements had a flood of unresolved emotions pulling in different directions. It was impossible for her to address all the problems but the dream indicated that she needed to take some action. Being aware and thinking about these complex issues was a starting point.

The second dream contained a high level of emotion, a person with bleeding teeth (whom she eventually recognised as herself), and the dreamer observing the scene. In making associations with 'bleeding teeth', she described first 'someone sick and dying', then pain, then her sister who had recently died of cancer. Her stream of associations continue, and she recounted how the circumstances of her sister's death were very painful, not only due to her illness but because of a very tragic background. The story had started eighteen years previously when her sister had the first of two children. She had confided to the patient that the child was not the son of her husband but was conceived during an affair with someone else. After a few years the sister told her husband, who left her, taking the second child with him. When she became ill with cancer, she was virtually alone and had no one to help her except the patient, who had been very close to her and had lived her emotional turmoil until she eventually died.

Both dreams were recurring and had strong emotional components of unhappiness and fear. Their content by association led to personal facts, which needed insight and would be unsettling for anyone. The dream content could be a fertile ground for psychoanalysis as an example of the dreamer disguising the truth by inverting the role in the first dream. Perhaps there could be an element of symbolism in the second. However, this approach would be very reductionist and of little use. It is much more informative to use the dream as the lead to unravelling the complex interaction of the underlying facts and emotions. Sometimes they can be the keys to a complex puzzle. No one else but the patient could 'interpret the dream'. Counsellors are only able to encourage insight and, perhaps, indicate a method of dream interpretation.

✳ Theories on the function of dreams

Psychoanalytic view of dreams

Freud's book *The Interpretation of Dreams* is a fundamental work on dreaming. Although his ideas have generated much controversy, and even hostility, Freud must be credited with having moved dreams from the mythical and divine world to more scientific ground. Allowing for the limited medical knowledge of his time, his ideas were very innovative. He worked mostly with patients suffering from neurosis (anxiety disorders and phobias), and his practice influenced his theory. He viewed dreams as the fulfilment of deep-seated wishes derived invariably, in his view, from childhood experiences and the sexual drive, either real facts or fantasy. Central to his thinking was the idea of *manifest* and *latent* dream content and the use of *symbols*. He would argue that what we recall as dreams (manifest content) is the result of elaboration of primitive forbidden wishes that can surface to consciousness only after they have been disguised (latent content) in order to avoid tension with moral principles. By preventing conflict between these wishes and the superego (moral principles), dreaming prevents a person from waking up. Therefore, dreams are considered the 'guardian of sleep'.

In Freud's view, symbols were a way to disguise sexual organs. So, anything with a sharp profile was interpreted as the equivalent of the male genitals, and cavities were often interpreted as symbols of the female genitals. The sensation of flying, floating or riding was interpreted as sexual activity, or the desire for it.

Another mechanism of disguise is *displacement*. This may involve swapping the identity of a person or a feeling. For example, it could be said that the first dream of the patient described above, where she is upset because the boyfriend has left her for another woman, is an example of displacement of person. In fact, in real life she had left the boyfriend, and not vice versa.

In order to reveal the latent content of dreams, Freud used the technique of *free association*. The value of free association in uncovering important personal issues is undisputed. However, Freud's view of dreams as childhood wishes and conflict was very restrictive and was criticised by other psychoanalysts. Carl Gustav Jung, for example, refused to trace dreams back to childhood experiences. He advised that dreams be taken at face value (the manifest content *is* the dream) with its own language of which symbols are a part. He considered current experiences a fundamental element of dreaming even though the dreaming mind may be tapping into previous life experiences, including childhood events.

Jung recognised that some emotional aspects of our inner life are common to everyone. The uncertainty of life and death, the tension between love and hate, God and Evil, and good and bad, are universal themes which he named *archetypes*. He postulated that, at times, our dreams reflect our personal ideas and emotions in regard to these topics.

Another aspect of Jung's theories is that dreams should be seen in series, rather than in isolation. If dreams are a form of 'thinking' during sleep, then their content is likely to be linked. Understanding one dream may help to clarify the meaning of another occurring at the same time.

These views, which depart from strict Freudian theory, were taken further by later psychoanalytic movements. Interpretation of dreams moved from patients with psychiatric illnesses to 'normal' people. Gestalt therapy, started by Frederick Perls, has been very popular. Analysis is conducted often in group sessions. Dreams are seen as a reflection of *current* ongoing aspects of the person. The dreamer is requested to personify the individual elements of the dream. In the example used above where the patient dreams of being left by her boyfriend for another woman, the dreamer would be requested to take the part of the boyfriend and to express his view on the matter. She would then be asked to personify and speak on behalf of the woman the boyfriend left her for, and so on. In this manner, the dreamer generates associations that are revealing of her thoughts and, at times, contrasting emotions. The Gestalt movement concentrates more on *using* dreams than on giving an explanation of their function.

Reverse learning theory

Reverse learning theory was put forward by Frances Crick and Graeme Mitchison, the former better known for his discovery of the elical structure of DNA. In very simple terms, they proposed that dreaming has the function of deleting superfluous information. The action of dreaming is similar to the de-fragmenting of the hard drive of a computer. In fact, their proposal draws from the computing concept of neural network (artificial intelligence) theories. Their proposal, put forward in 1983, still assumed that dreaming was predominantly a REM sleep activity. Therefore, the reverse learning hypothesis refers mostly to REM sleep.

Crick and Mitchison used their knowledge from anatomy that neurones (the nervous system cells) have multiple connections and that we learn by establishing specific patterns of links between them. Similarly, information in the hard drive of a computer is stored in particular units called clusters, which are interconnected and cross-linked. They reasoned that during the process of learning, incorrect or inefficient pattern connections may form. They called these *parasitic modes*.

Dreaming has the function of tuning up the links in the same manner as a de-fragmenting program cleans up a hard disk.

Dreams were the result of this process, they claimed. The computer-literate are familiar with files created when the hard drive is de-fragmented. These files often have a collage of information obtained from different files and make little sense. Similarly, our dreams contain bits and pieces from different parts of our mind and are only loosely associated, if at all.

The most important objection to this theory is that medications, which suppress REM sleep entirely, don't prevent learning. There is also some evidence that REM sleep, soon after information gathering, *consolidates* learning.

The genetic programming hypothesis

This theory was put forward by the French researcher Michel Jouvet and is more strictly linked to REM sleep, rather than to dreams as such. The background of Jouvet's idea is the growing evidence from studies of identical twins that personality traits depend on genetic as much as environmental factors. At brain level, a genetically determined personality trait is stored by connecting a network of cells according to a certain pattern (different patterns of connection for different traits). As well as aspects of our personality being determined by our genes, everyday life experiences also change the way we feel and behave and these changes are stored by continuously altering the nerve cell connections.

Jouvet hypothesised that periodic activation of the brain during REM sleep (every ninety minutes during sleep) has the function of re-programming nerve connections to maintain our psychological individuality. This activity would be genetically determined (coded in the genes we receive from our parents).

In general, theories on the *function* of dreams are influenced by current anatomical and physiological knowledge. As our understanding of brain organisation becomes more sophisticated, further theories closer to the truth will be developed.

However, the question of *why* we dream is much more difficult to answer because it goes beyond medicine and physiology and spills into the realm of philosophy, which attempts to answer questions such as 'Why do we think?' 'Why are we conscious?' and 'Why are we alive?'.

Appendix 1

Sleep-related internet sites

The following websites contain information on many aspects of sleep and wake function.

The Sleep Medicine Home Page
http://www.cloud9.net/~thorpy/
This page contains a wealth of information. You can find: sleep-related news and discussion groups, lots of links to other sleep pages, research sites and abstracts, text information files and an extensive coverage of sleep disorders. It contains a worldwide listing of sleep disorders centres.

The Sleep Home Page
http://bisleep.medsch.ucla.edu/
Contains a comprehensive resource for people interested in the research and treatment of sleep and sleep–wake disorders.

SleepNet
http://www.sleepnet.com/
Much information and over 168 links to other sleep pages.

The Sleep Well
http://www.stanford.edu/~dement/
A rich source of information for both professional and lay people interested in sleep disorders.

Newcastle Sleep Disorders Centre
http://www.newcastle.edu.au/department/md/sleep/
You can ask questions on sleep disorders through our website.

The American Association for Chronic Fatigue Syndrome
http://www.aacsf.org/
Information on chronic fatigue syndrome current research.

Association for Light Treatment and Biological Rhythms
http://www.websciences.org/sltbr
A source of information on light therapy.

Light Boxes
http://www.apollolight.com
http://lighttherapyproducts.com

Appendix 2

International sleep organisations

The World Federation of Sleep Research Societies maintains a database of sleep researchers and clinicians worldwide. It can be accessed at http://www.websciences.org/directory/default_alt.html

The following Sleep Societies also provide useful information on how to contact a sleep unit close to where you live:

American Sleep Disorders Association
1610 14th St NW, Suite 300
Rochester, MN 55901
Phone (507) 287 6006
Fax (507) 287 7008

Asian Sleep Research Society
http://www.WFSRS.org/iasrs.html

Australasian Sleep Association
http://www.WFSRS.org/iasa.html

British Sleep Society
PO Box 247
Huntingdon RE 17 3U2
United Kingdom

Canadian Sleep Society
3080 Yonge St Ste 5055
Toronto, ON
Canada
Phone (416) 483 6260
Fax (416) 483 7081

European Sleep Research Society
http://www.esrs.org/

Latino American Sleep Society
http://www.WFSRS.org/ilass.html

NODDS
Narcolepsy and Overwhelming Daytime
Sleep Society of Australasia
PO Box 100
Rosanna VIC 3084
(03) 9761 9767
(03) 9432 9669

Appendix 3

Sleep centres and support groups in Australasia

Australian Capital Territory

Canberra
Canberra Sleep Laboratory
(02) 6282 4955

New South Wales

Annandale
The Camperdown Sleep
Investigation Centre
(02) 9566 4044

Bondi Junction
Centre for Breathing Disorders
(02) 9387 6622

Camperdown
Royal Prince Alfred Hospital
(02) 9515 8876

RPAH Medical Centre
(02) 9565 1137

Coffs Harbour
Sleep Disorders Clinic
(02) 6652 7744

Port Maquarie Sleep Disorders
(02) 6583 6422

Concord
Concord Hospital Sleep Clinic
(02) 9767 7250

Darlinghurst
St Vincent's Hospital
(02) 9361 2330

St Vincent's Private Hospital
Sleep Investigation Centre
(02) 9332 6822

Hornsby
Sleep Disorders &
Diagnostic Centre
(02) 9476 5311

Kogarah
St George Hospital
Sleep Disorders Centre
(02) 9350 2696

Newcastle
Royal Newcastle Hospital
(02) 4923 6833

Warners Bay Private Hospital
(02) 4923 6833

Central Coast Respiratory
Services
(02) 4323 9988

Paediatric Sleep Units
Illawarra Sleep Disorders
Service
(Wollongong)
(02) 4226 6980

John Hunter Hospital
(Newcastle)
(02) 4921 3933

New Children's Hospital
(Sydney)
(02) 9845 3437

Sydney Children's Sleep Clinic
(02) 9314 7255

St Leonards
Royal North Shore Hospital
(02) 9926 8673

Sutherland
Sutherland Sleep Unit
(02) 9526 8222

Westmead
Charles Wentworth Hospital
(02) 9689 1133

Westmead Sleep Laboratory
(02) 9845 6042
(1.30 p.m.–7 a.m.)

Wollongong
Illawarra Sleep Disorders
Service
(02) 4226 6980
(02) 4227 1944

Tasmania

Hobart
Hobart Sleep Disorders Unit
(03) 6214 3041

Launceston
Mersey Community Hospital
Sleep Medicine Unit
(03) 6426 5111

Western Australia

Paediatric Sleep Unit
Princess Margaret Hospital
for Children
(08) 9340 8830

Perth
Sir Charles Gairdner Hospital
(08) 9346 2888

Subiaco
St John of God Hospital
(08) 9382 6111

South Australia

Adelaide
Royal Adelaide Hospital
(08) 8222 4000

Daw Park
Repatriation General Hospital
(08) 8276 9666

Paediatric Sleep Unit
Adelaide Children's Hospital
(08) 8204 7000

Toorak Gardens
Burnside Hospital Sleep Unit
(08) 8202 7272

Woodville South
The Queen Elizabeth Hospital
(08) 8222 6000

Queensland

Auchenflower
Wesley Hospital Sleep Unit
(07) 3870 2144

Buderim
Buderim Sleep Laboratory
(07) 5430 3303

Cairns
Calvary Hospital Sleep Unit
(07) 4052 5200

Chermside
Prince Charles Hospital
Sleep Unit
(07) 3350 8803

Everton Park
North West Hospital Sleep
Unit
(07) 3246 3103

Gold Coast
Gold Coast Sleep Disorders
(07) 5527 0555

Herston
Royal Brisbane Hospital
Sleep Unit
(07) 3253 7633

Mackay
Pioneer Valley Hospital
Sleep Unit
(07) 4942 1144

Paediatric Sleep Unit
Mater Hospital Children's
Unit (Brisbane)
(07) 3840 8078

Rockhampton
Mater Hospital Sleep
Unit
(07) 4931 3467

South Brisbane
Mater Private Hospital
Sleep Unit
(07) 3846 7955

Spring Hill
St Andrew's Hospital Sleep
Unit
(07) 3839 8608

Sunnybank
Sleep Unit
(07) 3344 4697

Toowoomba
St Andrew's Hospital Sleep
Unit
(07) 4631 4666

Townsville
Mater Private Sleep Unit
(07) 4725 3031

Woolloongabba
Princess Alexandra Sleep
Unit
(07) 3240 5147

Victoria

Ballarat
St John of God Hospital
(03) 5320 2392

Clayton
Monash Medical Centre
(03) 9550 2280

Fitzroy
St Vincent's Hospital
(03) 9288 3128

Footscray
Western General Hospital
(03) 9319 6842

Frankston
Frankston Hospital
(03) 9784 7050

Heidelberg
Austin & Repatriation
Medical Centre, Bowen House
(03) 9496 3688

Noble Park
South Eastern District Hospital
(03) 9549 6454

Paediatric Sleep Unit
Monash Medical Centre
(03) 9550 4488

Royal Children's Hospital
(03) 9345 6840

Parkville
Royal Melbourne Hospital
(03) 9342 8491

Prahran
Alfred Sleep Disorders Centre
(03) 9276 3770

Richmond
Epworth Hospital
(03) 9427 1849

New Zealand

Green Lane Hospital
Green Lane West
Auckland
(09) 638 9909

Christchurch Hospital
2 Riccarton Street
Christchurch
(03) 364 0640

Waikato Hospital
Pembroke Street
Hamilton
(07) 839 8899

Sleep Disorders Australia Branches

New South Wales
PO Box 303
Roseville 2069
(02) 9990 3514

Queensland
PO Box 1182
Coorparoo DC 4151
(07) 3378 1610

South Australia
PO Box 153
Kent Town 5071
(08) 8232 5319 (City)
1800 813 629 (Country)

Tasmania
PO Box 302
Mowbray 7248
(03) 6326 7889

Victoria
288 Springfield Rd
Nunawading 3131
(03) 9878 7145

Western Australia
36 Darley St
Bullcreek 6149
(08) 9332 1037

Appendix 4

The function of sleep

To satisfactorily answer the important question of why we sleep, requires a detailed understanding of the process of sleep. Our current knowledge allows us to give only a tentative answer.

From the previous chapters, you will have seen how sleep is divided into multiple states (stages)—REM and non-REM stages 1, 2, 3 and 4. Although this division is artificial, it highlights that sleep is a dynamic state likely to have *multiple functions*. I have also emphasised that sleep and wake are intimately linked, and are, in fact, aspects of a 24-hour cycle. Therefore any theory on the function of sleep will need to take into account the continuity of wakefulness and sleep.

As the cycling of sleep and wake is an universal phenomenon in animals, theory also needs to account for the evolutionary significance of sleep. If you were to look at sleep in isolation (not linked to wakefulness), it would seem to confer a survival disadvantage. Even allowing for the search for a secure place to sleep, an animal would still be vulnerable to attack by predators during sleep, when it is defenceless.

However, if sleep is seen as part of the sleep and wake cycle, it might actually provide a survival advantage. This would be the case if the highly sophisticated level of functioning during wakefulness was only possible due to the foundation laid during sleep.

Wakefulness behaviour is driven by instincts (for example hunger, thirst, flight or fight reaction) and by learned experience. Instincts provide the basic functions for survival, but it is learning and how learning modulates behaviour that provide the highest level of adaption and survival advantage.

Any explanation of the 'function' of sleep needs to take into consideration that sleep and wake are closely linked, and that sleep has a variety of states and therefore more than one function. None of the current theories satisfies these requirements.

✻ Rest-recovery theory

The observation that during sleep there is a reduction in motor activity, respiration, heart rate and temperature (to mention the most important physiological functions) makes the idea of sleep as a recovery period intuitive. This was the basis of the view that sleep is a resting period for the body to recover energy for the following day. However, the observation that REM sleep is a state of activation and that the growth hormone is specifically secreted during non-REM sleep makes the rest-recovery theory unsatisfactory and certainly an insufficient explanation of sleep. Moreover, if resting were the only function of sleep, it would be sufficient to stay inactive without the need to fall asleep, thus endangering safety.

Despite these considerations, it is still possible that sleep is needed to allow specific systems within the brain to be fully functional. It is hypothesised that the memory network and the systems, such as the one that handles all the sensory information (visual, auditory, body feelings and body position) we receive when awake, use specific molecules (proteins) during the day and accumulate them again during sleep.

✻ REM sleep related theory of sleep

The discovery of REM sleep in the early 1950s, and the observation that it is a state of brain activation, has generated a hypothesis that sleep is an active functional state.

The *learning theory* suggests that during REM sleep information aquired during the day and temporarily stored in memory is consolidated. It is believed that information is stored in the brain by creating patterns of connection between neurones (cells of the nervous system). Different patterns are created for different information. During REM sleep these connections are reinforced and memory is thus consolidated. The observation that learning is improved when information is gathered before REM sleep may support this theory. How this happens in practice is a subject of speculation. However, the learning theory does *not* refer to the popular belief that people can learn during sleep (sleep learning). It would be handy, but it does not happen!

A variant of the learning theory is the *reverse learning hypothesis* which also focuses on REM sleep and is discussed in Chapter 10.

The observation that REM sleep is the predominant state in the foetus and in infants has led to the suggestion that REM sleep is needed to imprint behaviours that are already present at birth and are needed for survival. Newborns coordinate their muscles to breathe a few seconds after birth and can start sucking to be fed immediately. The hypothesis is that the foetus is prepared for these activities during active sleep (REM sleep). A similar role for REM sleep in adults has been put forward in the genetic programming hypothesis by Michael Jouvet (see Chapter 10).

It can be said that no single theory or set of theories adequately explains the function of sleep. Its may well be that all the theories put forward so far are correct in some way, as they identify different functions of sleep. With more knowledge other functions will be discovered.

Further reading

Chapter 1 An overview of sleep

Carskadon, M.A. and Dement, W.C. 1992 'Nocturnal determinants of daytime sleepiness' *Sleep* no. 5, pp. 573–81.

French, J.D. 1957 'The reticular formation' *Scientific American* vol. 196, no. 5, pp. 54–60.

Gale, C. and Martyn, C. 1998 'Larks and owls and health, wealth, and wisdom' *BMJ (Clinical Research Ed)* vol. 317, no. 7174, pp. 1675–7.

Kryger, M.H., Roth, T. and Carskadon, M. 1994 'Circadian rhythm in humans: An overview in principle and practice of sleep medicine' *Principles and Practice of Sleep Medicine* 2nd edn, eds M.H. Kryger, T. Roth and W.C. Dement, Saunders, Philadelphia.

Monk, T. and Folkard, S. 1976 'Adjusting to the changes to and from daylight saving time' *Nature* vol. 261, pp. 688–9.

Parkes, J.D. 1985 'Circadian rhythms and sleep' *Sleep and its Disorders* ed. J.D. Parkes, W.B. Saunders, London.

——1985 'Normal sleep, its variants and related states' *Sleep and its Disorders* ed. J.D. Parkes, W.B. Saunders, London.

Roffwarg, H.P., Muzio, J.N. and Dement, W.C. 1966 'Ontogenic development of the human sleep–dream cycle' *Science* vol. 152, pp. 604–19.

Youngstadt, S.D., Kripke, DF and Elliott, J.A., 1999 'Is sleep disturbed by vigorous late night exercise?' *Medicine and Science in Sports and Exercise* vol. 31, no. 6, pp. 864–9.

Chapter 2 How sleep is measured

American Sleep Disorders Association 1992 'The clinical use of the multiple sleep latency test'. *Sleep* vol. 15, pp. 268–76.

Gyulay, S.G., Olson, L.G., Hensley, M.J., King, M.A.T., Murree-Allen, K. and Saunders, N.A. 1993 'Comparison of clinical assessment and home oximetry in the diagnosis of obstructive sleep apnoea' *American Review of Respiratory Disorders* vol. 147, pp. 50–53.

Johns, M.W. 1991 'A new method for measuring daytime sleepiness: The Epworth Sleepiness Scale' *Sleep*, vol. 14, pp. 540–5.

Morin, C.M. 1993 *Insomnia* The Guilford Press, New York, p. 210.

The Thoracic Society of Australia and New Zealand July 1990 *Guidelines for Respiratory Sleep Studies* Fellowship Affairs, pp. 16–18.

Chapter 3   Snoring and disturbed breathing

Bearpark, H., Elliott, L., Grunstein, R.R., Cullen, S., Schneider, H., Althaus, W. and Sullivan, C. 1995 'Snoring and sleep apnoea: A population study in Australian men' *American Review of Respiratory and Critical Care Medicine* vol. 151, pp. 1459–65.

Cistulli, P.A. and Sullivan, C.E. 1993 'Sleep-disordered breathing in Marfan's syndrome', *American Review of Respiratory and Critical Care Medicine*, vol. 147, pp. 645–8.

Ferber, R. and Kryger, M. 1995 *Principles and Practice of Sleep Medicine in the Child*, Saunders, Philadelphia.

Friberg, D., Carlsson-Nordlander, B., Larsson, H. and Svamborg, E. 1995 'UPPP for habitual snoring: A 5 years follow-up with respiratory sleep recording' *Laryngoscope* vol. 105, pp. 519–22.

Grunstein, R.R., Ellis, E., Hillman, D., McEvoy, R.D., Robertson, C.F. and Saunders, N.A. 1991 'Treatment of sleep disordered breathing', *Medical Journal of Australia*, vol. 154, pp. 355–9.

Guilleminault, C. and Stoohs, R. 1990 'Upper airway resistance syndrome' *Sleep Research* vol. 1991, pp. 20:250.

Hoffstein, V.V. 1996 'Snoring' *Chest* vol. 108, pp. 201–22.

Joel-Cohen, S.J. and Schoenfeld, A. 1978 'Fetal responses to periodic sleep apnoea: A new syndrome in obstetrics' *European Journal of Obstetrics, Gynecology and Reproduction Biology*, vol. 8, no. 2, pp. 77–81.

Kryger, M.H. 1993 'Snoring: A public health hazard?' *Chest* vol. 104, pp. 2–3.

Loube, D.L., Poceta, J.S., Morales, M.C., Peacock, M.D. and Mitler, M.M. 1996 'Self-reported snoring in pregnancy. Association with fetal outcome' *Chest* vol. 109, no. 4, pp. 859–61.

Olson, L.G., King, M.T., Hensley, M.J. and Saunders, N.A. 1995 'A community study of snoring and sleep-disordered breathing prevalence'

American Review of Respiratory and Critical Care Medicine, vol. 52, pp. 711–16.

Saunders, N.A., Vandeleur, T., Deves, J., Salmon, A., Gyulay, S., Crocker, B. and Hensley, M. 1989 'Uvulopalatopharyngoplasty as treatment for snoring', *Medical Journal of Australia*, vol. 150, pp. 177–82.

Chapter 4 Body jerks and restless limbs

Ambrogetti, A., Olson, L.G. and Saunders, N.A. 1991 'Disorders of movement and behaviour during sleep' *Medical Journal of Australia*, vol. 155, pp. 336–40.

American Sleep Disorders Association 1997 *The International Classification of Sleep Disorders* pp. 142–68.

Lansky, M.R. and Bley, R. 1995 *Nightmares. Psychodynamic exploration*, The Analytic Press, London.

Meierkord, H. 1994 'Epilepsy and sleep' *Current Opinion in Neurology* vol. 7, pp. 107–12.

Montplaisir, J., Lapierre, O., Warnes, H. and Pellettier, G. 1992 'The treatment of the restless leg syndrome with or without periodic limb movement in sleep' *Sleep vol. 15, no. 5, pp. 391–5.*

Provini, F., Plazzi, G., Tinuper, P. et al. 1999 'Nocturnal frontal lobe epilepsy' *Brain* vol. 122, pp. 1017–31.

Schenk, C.H., Bundle, S.R., Ettinger, M.G. and Mahowald, M.W. 1986 'Chronic behavioural disorders of human REM sleep: A new category of parasomnia' *Sleep* vol. 9, no. 2, pp. 293–308.

Chapter 5 Insomnia

American Sleep Disorders Association 1997 *The International Classification of Sleep Disorders Diagnostic and Coding Manual* pp. 27–38.

Buysse, D.J. and Reynold III, C.F. 1990 'Insomnia' Thorpy MJ edition. *Handbook of Sleep Disorders* ed. M.J. Thorpy, Marcel Dekker, New York.

Houri, P. and Fisher, J. 1986 'Persistent psychophysiological (learned) insomnia' *Sleep* no. 1, pp. 38–53.

Houri, P. and Esther, M.S. 1990 'Insomnia', *Mayo Clin. Prac.* vol. 65, pp. 868–82.

Morin, C.M. and Esther, M.S. 1993 *Insomnia. Psychological Assessment and Management*, The Guilford Press, New York.

Sleep Disorders and Insomnia in the Elderly 1993 *Facts and Research in Gerontology* vol. 7.

Standards of Practice Committee of the American Sleep Disorders Association 1995 'Practice parameters for the use of polysomnography in the evaluation of insomnia' *Sleep* vol. 18, no. 1, pp. 55–57.

Chapter 6   Sleepiness, tiredness and fatigue

Akerstedt, T. 1988 'Sleepiness as a consequence of shift work' *Sleep* vol. 11, no. 1, pp. 17–34.

Akerstedt, T., Torsvall, L. and Gillberg, M. 1982 'Sleepiness and shift work: field studies' *Sleep* vol. 5, pp. S95–S106.

Akerstedt, T., Torsvall, L. and Gillberg, M. 1988 'Shift work and napping' *Sleep and Alertness* eds David F. Dinges and Roger J. Broughton, Raven Press, New York.

Ambrogetti, A. and Olson, L.G. 1994 'Consideration of narcolepsy in the differential diagnosis of chronic fatigue syndrome' *Medical Journal of Australia,* vol. 160, pp. 426–8.

Arendt, J., Skene, D.J., Midleton, B., Lockley, S.W. and Deacon, S. 1997 'Efficacy of melatonin treatment in jet lag, shift work and blindness' *Journal of Biological Rhythms* vol. 12, no. 6, pp. 604–17.

Carskadon, M.A. and Dement, W.C. 1982 'Nocturnal determinants of daytime sleepiness' *Sleep* vol. 5, pp. 573–81.

Chronic Fatigue Syndrome. Working Group, Royal Australasian College of Physicians. 1997 (http://www.mja.com.au/public/guides/cfs/cfs1.htm1).

Eastman, C.I. 1990 'Circadian rhythms and bright light: Recommendations for shift work' *Work and Stress* vol. 4, no. 3, pp. 245–60.

Jenkins, R. and Mowbray, J. 1991 *Post-viral Fatigue Syndrome* John Wiley and Sons, Chichester.

Kroenke, K., Wood, D.R., Mangelsdorff, A.D., Meier, N.J. and Powell, J.B. 1988 'Chronic fatigue in primary care. Prevalence, patients' characteristics and outcome' *JAMA* vol. 260, pp. 929–34.

Lugaresi, E., Montagna, P., Tinuper, P. et al. 1998 'Endozepine stupor. Recurring stupor linked to endozepine–4 accumulation' *Brain* vol. 121, pp. 127–33.

Mitler, M.M., Aldrich, M.S., Kacob, G.F. and Zarcone, V.P. 1994 'Narcolepsy and its treatment with stimulants' *Sleep* vol. 17, no. 4, pp. 312–71.

Pearn, J.H. 1997 'Chronic fatigue syndrome: chronic ciguatera poisoning as a differential diagnosis' *Medical Journal of Australia* vol. 166, 308–10.

Pilcher, J.J. and Huffcutt, A.I. 1996 'Effects of sleep deprivation on performance: A meta analysis' *Sleep* vol. 19, no. 4, pp. 318–26.

Roth, B. 1980 *Narcolepsy and Hypersomnia* Karger S, Basel.

Standards of Practice Committee of the American Sleep Disorder Association 1994 'Practice parameters for the use of stimulants in the treatment of narcolepsy' *Sleep* vol. 17, no. 4, pp. 348–51.

Totterdell, P., Spelten, E., Smith, L., Barton, J. and Falkard, S. 1995 'Recovery from work shifts: How long does it take?' *Journal of Applied Psychology* vol. 80, no. 1, pp. 43–57.

Tucker, P., Barton, J. and Folkard, S. 1996 'Comparison of eight and twelve hour shifts: Impacts on health, well being and alertness during the shift' *Occupational and Environmental Medicine* vol. 53, pp. 767–72.

Utley, M.J. 1995 *Narcolepsy. A Funny Disorder That's Not a Laughing Matter* M.J. Utley, PO Box 1923, Desoto, TX 75123–1923 USA.

Chapter 7   Children and sleep

Anders, T., Halpern, L. and Hua, J. 1992 'Sleeping through the night: Origin in early infancy' *Pediatrics* vol. 90, pp. 554–60.

Anders, T. and Keener, M. 1985 'Developmental course of nighttime sleep–wake patterns in full term and premature infants in the first year of life' *Sleep* vol. 8, pp. 173–92.

Bernal, J. 1973 'Night waking in infants during the first fourteen months' *Developmental Medicine and Child Neurology* vol. 15, pp. 760–9.

Carroll, J.L. and Loughlin, G.M. 1995 'Primary Snoring in Children' *Principles and Practice of Sleep Medicine in the Child* eds Ferber, R. and Kryger, M., Saunders, Philadelphia.

——1995 'Obstructive Sleep Apnea Syndrome in Infants and Children: Diagnosis and Management' *Principles and Practice of Sleep Medicine in the Child* eds Ferber, R. and Kryger, M. Saunders, Philadelphia.

France, K.G. and Hudson, S.M. 1993 'Management of infant sleep disturbance: A review' *Clinical Psychology Review* vol. 23, pp. 635–47.

Chapter 8   Medications and sleep

Brzezinski, A. 1997 'Mechanisms of disease: Melatonin in humans', *New England Journal of Medicine* vol. 16, no. 3, pp. 186–95.

Fleming, J.E. 1997 'Pharmacological Aspects of Drowsiness' *Forensic Aspects of Sleep* eds C. Shapiro and A. McCall Smith, John Wiley and Sons, Chichester.

Holmes, V.F. 1995 'Medical use of psychostimulant: An overview' *International Psychiatry in Medicine* vol. 25, no. 1, pp. 1–19.

Mendelson, W.B. 1997 'A clinical evaluation of the hypnotic efficacy of melatonin' *Sleep* vol. 20, no. 10, pp. 916–19.

Mitler, M.M. and Hajdukovic R. 1991 'Relative efficacy of drugs for the treatment of sleepiness in narcolepsy' *Sleep* vol. 14 pp. 218–20.

US Modafinil in Narcolepsy Study Group 1998 'Randomized trial of Modafinil for the treatment of pathological somnolence in narcolepsy' *Annals of Neurology* vol. 43, pp. 88–97.

Zhdanova, I.V., Lynch, H.J. and Wurtman, R.O. 1997 'Melatonin: A sleep promoting hormone' *Sleep* vol. 20, no. 10, pp. 899–907.

Chapter 9   Sleep disorders and driving

Aldrich, M.S. 1989 'Automobile accidents in patients with sleep disorders' *Sleep* vol. 12, no. 6, pp. 487–94.

Assessing Fitness to Drive 1988 Austroads, Sydney.

Dawson, D. Reid, K. 1997 'Fatigue, alcohol and performance impairment' *Nature* vol. 388, p. 235.

Fell, D. 1994 *Screening of truck drivers for sleep apnoea in New South Wales: Potential road safety benefit in Stay Safe 28* New South Wales Parliament Joint Standing Committee on Road Safety, December.

Medical Examination of Commercial Vehicle Drivers 1994 National Road Transport Commission.

Mitler, M.M., Carskadon, M.A., Czeisler, C.A., Dement, W.C., Dinges, D.F. and Graeber, R.C. 1988 'Catastrophes, sleep and public policy' *Sleep* vol. 11, pp. 100–9.

Pack, A.I., Pakola, S.J., and Findley, L.J. 1997 'Regulation for Driving for Patients with Sleep Disorders' *Forensic Aspects of Sleep Disorders* eds C. Shapiro and A. McCall Smith, John Wiley and Sons, Chichester.

Chapter 10   Dreams and dreaming

Aserinsky, E. and Kleitman, N. 1995 'Two types of ocular motility occurring in sleep' *Journal of Applied Physiology* vol. 8, no. 1, July, pp. 1–10.

Berger, R.J., Olley, P. and Oswald, I. 1962 'The EEG, eye-movements and dreams of the blind' *Quarterly Journal of Experimental Psychology* vol. 14, pp. 183–6.

Crick, F. and Mitchison, G. 1983 'The function of dream sleep' *Nature* vol. 304, July, pp. 111–14.

Dement, W. and Wolpert, E.A., 1958 'The relation of eye movements, body motility, and external stimuli to dream content' *Journal of Experimental Psychology* vol. 55, no. 6, pp. 543–53.

Faraday, A. 1997 *Dream Power* Berkley Publishing, Berkley, New York.

Foulkes, D. 1982 *Children's Dreams: Longitudinal Studies* Wiley, New York.

Jouvet, M. 1999 *The Paradox of Sleep* A Bradford Book, The MIT Press, Cambridge, Massachussetts.

Ladd, G.T. 1892 'Contribution to the physiology of visual dreams' *Mind* vol. 2, April, pp. 299–304.

Padgham, C.A. 1975 'Colours experienced in dreams' *British Journal of Psychology* vol. 66, no. 1, pp. 25–8.

Glossary

Achondroplasia Disease of cartilage and bone development which results in small stature (dwarf)

Adenoidectomy Surgical removal of the adenoids

Advanced sleep phase syndrome Disorder of the sleep/wake timing. People with this disorder tend to go to sleep early in the evening and wake up in the early hours of the morning. They complain of difficulty maintaining sleep (that is, they wake too early).

Apnoea Stopping breathing completely

Atrophy Diminution in size and usual function of any organ or part or the body; for example, the liver shrinks in cirrhosis (liver atrophy).

Benzodiazepine Medications widely used as sleeping tablets and anti-anxiety medication. Among the many benzodiazepine Valium™ is widely known.

Brain stem Part of the brain between the cerebral hemisphere (cortex) and the spinal cord. It is the most primitive of the brain present in all animals.

CT Computerised tomography

Cataplexy First to sudden onset of muscle weakness (jelly feeling) which can involve the entire body or an individual muscle. If it affects the knees, a person can have a sensation of knee buckling or may even fall on the ground without loss of consciousness.

Ciguatera Medical condition contracted by eating fish from tropical and sub-tropical areas that contain cigua toxin

Computerised tomography Radiology technique helpful to visualise internal organs (e.g. the brain)

Conversion syndrome Another word for hysteria, where psychic symptoms are *converted* into a body complaint. An example is anxiety that presents as shortness of breath.

Delayed sleep phase syndrome A sleep–wake function timing disorder characterised by inability to fall asleep until the early hours of the morning (past midnight) and a tendency to continue sleeping until late in the morning. Patients present with difficulty initiating sleep and daytime tiredness.

dopamine   A substance used by brain cells to communicate with each other (neurotransmitter)

Eckbom syndrome   Another name for restless leg syndrome after the researcher who initially described the symptoms

EEG   Electroencephalogram

Electroencephalogram   A technique for recording electrical brain activity

Encephalitis   Inflammation of the central nervous system (the brain) usually due to viruses or bacteria

Endorphin   Substance produced by the brain that helps reduce pain; 'body-own pain killers'

Endozepine   Substances produced by the nervous system that promote sleep

Entrainment   The coupling of two rhythms; for example, body temperature with sleep and wake function

Enuresis   Bed-wetting

Epoch   Recording of sleep parameters (brain activity, eye movement cardiograph and muscle tone) in 20–30 seconds periods

Fibromyalgia   Condition of chronic fatigue and diffuse aches and pains in the absence of inflammation in the muscle joints

Fibrositis   See fibromyalgia

Flumazenil   Medication that counteracts the action of benzodiazepine

Hallucinations   Perception of sensory experiences (seeing things, hearing things, feeling of abnormal body position) in the absence of a real stimulus

Hypersomnia   Increased tendency to sleepiness

Hypersomnolence   Another word for increased tendency to sleepiness

Hypnagogic hallucinations   Hallucinations that occur at the beginning of sleep (hypnagogic)

Hypnopompic hallucinations   Hallucinations that occur at the end of sleep (hypnopompic)

Hypopnoea   Reduction in breathing, contrary to apnoea which is stopping breathing completely

Hypothalamus   Part of the brain located at the top of the brain stem which, among other things, is involved in regulation of hormone secretion

Hypothyroidism   Condition characterised by reduction in the level of thyroid hormone

Hysteria   A word for conversion syndrome, but currently not used in psychiatry

Idiopathic   Medical word meaning 'of unknown origin', e.g. idiopathic hypersomnolence means increased sleepiness (hypersomnolence is of unknown origin)

Kleine-Levin syndrome   A condition characterised by compulsive eating and recurrent bouts of sleepiness lasting days to weeks

Limbic system   Part of the brain involved in the regulation of memory, concentration and emotion

M.E.   See Myalgic encephalitis

Magnetic resonance imaging   A radiological technique that uses a magnetic field to visualise internal body parts. It allows visualisation of the brain in fine detail.

Melatonin   Hormone produced in the brain by the pineal gland. It helps to synchronise the sleep–wake function with light and dark cycles.

MRI   See magnetic resonance imaging

Myalgic encephalitis   Term used for people with chronic fatigue. It implies, but never demonstrated, diffuse aches (myalgic) due to inflammation of the brain (encephalomyelitis).

Narcolepsy   A condition characterised by increased tendency to fall asleep

Neuro-asthenia   Name used for people with chronic fatigue. Literally it means weakness (asthenia) of the nervous system.

Neurone(s)   Cells in the nervous system

Neuropathy   Diseases of the peripheral nerves that can result in unpleasant sensations in the part of the body supplied by the nerve. It is very common in diabetes when it can cause numbness, tingling and pain, particularly in the legs.

Non-REM   Non-rapid eye movement sleep

Non-REM narcolepsy   A condition characterised by an increased sleepiness tendency with no evidence of rapid eye movement related symptoms (cataplexy, hallucinations and sleep paralysis)

Nor-adrenaline   A substance that is used by brain cells to communicate with each other (neuro-transmitter). It increases alertness.

Occipital cortex   Part of the brain cortex underneath the back of the skull. It is responsible for vision.

Ondine curse   Particular form of *central* sleep apnoea (see text).

Periodic limb movement disorder   A sleep disorder characterised by recurrent fast jerks of the ankles, knees, hips or arms during sleep. It causes sleep fragmentation, daytime tiredness and unrefreshed sleep. It is one of the causes of insomnia.

Pickwickian syndrome A condition characterised by obesity, apnoea, respiratory failure and daytime sleepiness. The name is derived from one of Charles Dickens' characters in *Pickwick Papers*.

Pineal gland Small gland in the brain that produces melatonin during darkness. It derives its name from its *pine* cone-like shape.

PLMD Periodic limb movement disorder

Polysomnography Recording of multiple (poly) parameters during sleep (somnography)

Psycho-asthenia A name used for people with chronic fatigue, literally meaning weakness (asthenia) of the psyche (soul)

REM Rapid eye movement

REM sleep behaviour disorder A sleep disorder characterised by acting out dreams during sleep

Restless leg A condition characterised by sensation of cramps in the calves. It usually occurs at bedtime and causes the need to move the legs around to relieve the discomfort.

Reticular activating system A group of neurones (cells of the nervous system) in the brain stem linked together like a net. They are active during wakefulness.

Retina Light sensitive layer of cells in the back of the eye where light and outside world images are registered

Sleep paralysis Sensation of not being able to move (paralysis) usually experienced when waking up. Lasting from a few seconds to a few minutes, it is a frightening experience.

Snoring The sound made by the air passing through the pharynx (the back of the throat) during sleep

Synchroniser An agent, such as melatonin or light, which determines the periodicity of a biological function. For example, light and darkness cycles synchronise our sleep and wake function. Synchronisers are also know as *zeitgeber* (time givers) or entraining agents.

Tonsillectomy Surgical removal of the tonsils

Upper airway resistance syndrome A condition halfway between pure snoring and sleep apnoea. Breathing does not stop completely because the body makes an extra effort to drive the air through the narrow pharynx. This results in fragmentation of sleep.